Health Promotion and Wellness

First Edition

Written and Edited by

JESSICA MAUREEN HARRIS, ED.D.,CHES

SUNY - Oswego

ELIZABETH KEIDA, ED.D.

SUNY - Oswego

AMY BIDWELL, PHD.

SUNY - Oswego

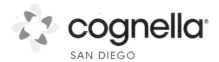

cognella®

SAN DIEGO

Bassim Hamadeh, CEO and Publisher
John Remington, Executive Editor
Tony Paese, Project Editor
Abbey Hastings, Production Editor
Emely Villavicencio, Senior Graphic Designer
Stephanie Kohl, Licensing Coordinator
Natalie Piccotti, Director of Marketing
Kassie Graves, Vice President of Editorial
Jamie Giganti, Director of Academic Publishing

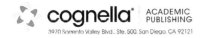 cognella® | ACADEMIC PUBLISHING

3970 Sorrento Valley Blvd., Ste. 500, San Diego, CA 92121

Brief Contents

Chapter 1   An Invitation to Health Promotion   1

Chapter 2   The Eight Dimensions of Wellness   12

Chapter 3   Historical Health and Its Influence on Wellness   23

Chapter 4   Investigation of Health Status   42

Chapter 5   The New Role of Information Technology in Health and Wellness   55

Chapter 6   A Background to Theory and Planning Models in Health Education and Promotion   67

Chapter 7   Improving and Implementing Health Promotion Through Cultural Competence   84

Chapter 8   Achieving Wellness Through Philosophy   95

Chapter 9   Ethics and Professionalism in Health Education and Health Promotion   106

Chapter 10   The Health Education Specialist   119

Chapter 11   Various Career Venues Related to Health Promotion and Wellness   134

Appendix A: Code of Ethics for the Health Education Profession Preamble   151

Appendix B: Areas of Responsibility, Competencies and Sub-Competencies for Health Education Specialist Practice Analysis II 2020 (HESPA II 2020)   156

Glossary   167

Index   177

Contents

Chapter 1   **An Invitation to Health Promotion**   **1**

Chapter Objectives   1
Chapter Links to the Areas of Responsibility of a Health Educator/Health Promotion Professional   2
Introduction   2
The Terminology of Health Education, Health Promotion, and Wellness   2
The Development of Health Education, Health Promotion, and Wellness   4
    Health Education   4
    Health Promotion   4
    Relationship Between Health Education and Health Promotion   5
Concepts and Practice of Health Promotion   6
The Goals and Purpose of the Profession   7
Summary   7
Review Questions   8
Case Scenario   8
Critical Thinking Questions   8
Activities   8
Web Links   9
References   10

Chapter 2   **The Eight Dimensions of Wellness**   **12**

Chapter Objectives   12
Chapter Links to the Areas of Responsibility of a Health Educator/Health Promotion Professional   12
Introduction   13
    Wellness   13
The Illness-Wellness Continuum   13
The Eight Dimensions of Wellness   14
    Emotional Wellness   14
    Environmental Wellness   15
    Financial Wellness   16
    Intellectual Wellness   16
    Physical Wellness   17
    Occupational Wellness   18

Social Wellness   18
Spiritual Wellness   19
Summary   19
Review Questions   20
Case Scenario   20
Critical Thinking Questions   20
Activities   21
Web Links   21
References   22

Chapter 3   **Historical Health and Its Influence on Wellness**   23

Chapter Objectives   23
Chapter Links to the Areas of Responsibility of a Health Educator/Health Promotion Professional   24
Introduction   24
Public Health   24
Evidence of Public Health in Early Cultures   24
Health Promotion and Wellness in Early Cultures   24
Middle Ages (500–1500)   25
Renaissance (1500–1700)   26
Age of Enlightenment (1700–1800)   27
The 1800s   27
Public Health Efforts in the United States   28
The 1700s   28
The 1800s   29
The 1900s   31
The 2000s to Present   35
A Recognized Profession   35
Summary   36
Review Questions   37
Case Study Scenario   37
Critical Thinking Questions   37
Activities   37
Web Links   38
References   39

Chapter 4   **Investigation of Health Status**   42

Chapter Objectives   42
Chapter Links to the Areas of Responsibility of a Health Educator/Health Promotion Professional   43
Introduction   43
Measuring Health Status   43

Rates   44
Leading Causes of Death   46
Healthy People 2030   46
The Levels of Prevention   47
Chain of Infection for Communicable Diseases   48
Multicausation Disease Model for Noncommunicable Diseases   49
Summary   50
Review Questions   50
Case Scenario   50
Critical Thinking Questions   51
Activities   51
Web Links   52
References   53

Chapter 5   The New Role of Information Technology in Health and Wellness   55

Chapter Objectives   55
Chapter Links to the Areas of Responsibility of a Health Educator/Health Promotion Professional   56
Introduction   56
How Technology Shapes Us   56
Mobile Devices and Social Media in Health Promotion   57
Smartphones and Apps That Motivate Change   58
Physical   58
Emotional, Spiritual, and Intellectual   59
Financial   60
Occupational and Social   60
Wearable Technology and Other Information   61
Telemedicine   61
Telehealth   62
Technology Trends in Healthcare and HIPPA   62
Review Questions   63
Case Scenario   63
Critical Thinking Questions   63
Activities   64
Weblinks   64
References   65

Chapter 6   A Background to Theory and Planning Models in Health Education and Promotion   67

Chapter Objectives   67
Chapter Links to the Areas of Responsibility of a Health Educator/Health Promotion Professional   68

Introduction   68
Primary Elements   68
The Importance of Theory and Planning Models   69
Behavior Change Theories   69
Intrapersonal Theories   69
  The Health Belief Model   69
  The Transtheoretical Model (Stages of Change)   71
  Theory of Planned Behavior   72
Interpersonal Theories   73
  Social Cognitive Theory   73
Community Theories   74
  Diffusion of Innovation Theory   74
  Community Readiness Model   75
Socio-Ecological Approach   76
Planning Models for Health Promotion and Wellness   77
  Generalized Model   77
  PRECEDE-PROCEED Model   78
Summary   80
Review Questions   80
Case Scenario   80
Critical Thinking Questions   80
Activity   81
Web Links   81
References   82

Chapter 7   **Improving and Implementing Health Promotion Through Cultural Competence**   **84**

Chapter Objectives   84
Chapter Links to the Areas of Responsibility of a Health Educator/Health Promotion Professional   85
Introduction   85
Importance of Cultural Competence   85
Involving All Stakeholders in the Process   86
Acquiring Cultural Competence   88
Ensuring Cultural Competence in Data Collection   89
Creating Positive Relationships   89
Summary   91
Review Questions   91
Case Scenario   92
Critical Thinking Questions   92
Activities   92

Web Links   93
References   94

Chapter 8   **Achieving Wellness Through Philosophy**   **95**

Chapter Objectives   95
Chapter Links to the Areas of Responsibility of a Health Educator/Health Promotion Professional   96
Introduction   96
Philosophy   96
The Importance of a Personal Philosophy for Health Educators   98
Philosophies Associated with Health and Wellness   99
Predominant Health Philosophies   100
Developing Your Own Health Philosophy   101
Summary   103
Review Questions   103
Case Scenario   104
Critical Thinking Questions   104
Activities   104
Weblinks   105
References   105

Chapter 9   **Ethics and Professionalism in Health Education and Health Promotion**   **106**

Chapter Objectives   106
Chapter Links to the Areas of Responsibility of a Health Educator/Health Promotion Professional   107
Introduction   107
The Terminology of Ethics   107
Health Educators' Ethical Areas of Responsibility   108
How Does Ethics Affect Our Health?   110
Ethical Principles   111
Ethical Theories   111
How to Make Ethical Decisions   113
Ethical Issues in Health Education and Health Promotion   114
Summary   114
Review Questions   115
Case Scenario   115
Critical Thinking Questions   115
Activities   115
Web Links   116
References   117

Chapter 10   The Health Education Specialist   119

Chapter Objectives   119
Chapter Links to the Areas of Responsibility of a Health Educator/Health Promotion Professional   120
Introduction   120
Who Are Health Educators?   120
    Certified Health Education Specialist or Health Educator   120
How to Become a Certified Health Education Specialist   121
Areas of Responsibility of a Health Educator   121
    Responsibility I: Assessment of Needs and Capacity   122
    Responsibility II: Planning   125
    Responsibility III: Implementation   126
    Responsibility IV: Evaluation and Research   127
    Responsibility V: Administer and Manage Health Education/Promotion   128
    Responsibility VI: Advocacy   129
    Responsibility VII: Communication   129
    Responsibility VIII: Ethics and Professionalism   130

Summary   130
Review Questions   130
Case Scenario   131
Critical Thinking Questions   131
Activities   131
Weblinks   132
References   132

Chapter 11   Various Career Venues Related to Health Promotion and Wellness   134

Chapter Objectives   134
Chapter Links to the Areas of Responsibility of a Health Educator/Health Promotion Professional   135
Introduction   135
Career Opportunities and Responsibilities of Health Educators   135
Careers for Health Educators and Health Promotion Specialists   136
    School Health Education   136
    Academia and University Health Education   136
    Community Health Education   137
    Business and Non-Profit Health Education   137
    Government and Health Departments   138
Skills and Qualities Employers Seek in Health Educators   139
    Technical Skills   139
    Transferable Skills   139
Job Search Strategies   140
    Self-Assessment and Exploring Career Options   140

Making Professional Connections   142
Preparing Job Search Materials   142
Getting Experience   143
Job Searching   143

Advanced Study and Applying to Graduate Schools   144
Common Choices for Master's Degree Programs and Post-Secondary Certifications   145
Professional Studies in Medicine and Healthcare   145
Graduate Admissions Requirements   146

Summary   146
Review Questions   146
Case Scenario   147
Critical Thinking Questions   147
Activities   147
Weblinks   148
References   150

Appendix A: Code of Ethics for the Health Education Profession Preamble   151

Article I: Responsibility to the Public   151
Article II: Responsibility to the Profession   152
Article III: Responsibility to Employers   153
Article IV: Responsibility in the Delivery of Health Education   153
Article V: Responsibility in Research and Evaluation   154
Article VI: Responsibility in Professional Preparation   155
Appendix B: Areas of Responsibility, Competencies and Sub-Competencies for Health Education Specialist Practice Analysis II 2020 (Hespa II 2020)   156

Glossary   167

Index   177

CHAPTER 1

An Invitation to Health Promotion

CHAPTER KEY

Authentic Learning: **using problem-solving of real-life scenarios to explore and discuss content and concepts.**

Collaboration: **working with content from other organizations or peers.**

Knowledge: **the theoretical or practical understanding of a concept.**

Practice: **applications of ideas or concepts.**

Reflection: **contemplation and meditation.**

Chapter Objectives

Upon completion of this chapter and participating in the critical thinking questions at the end, you should be able to master the following:

- **Differentiate** between keywords, terms, and definitions that promote health and health promotion (*knowledge and reflection*).

- **Explain** health promotion and wellness as "emerging professions" (*knowledge and reflection*).

- **Describe** the current status of health promotion and wellness (*knowledge, reflection, practice, and collaboration*).

- **Describe** the ultimate goal of health promotion (*authentic learning, reflection, practice, and collaboration*).

- **Explain** and **identify** the main concepts and priorities of health promotion (*authentic learning, reflection, practice, and collaboration*).

Chapter Links to the Areas of Responsibility of a Health Educator/Health Promotion Professional

- Area of Responsibility I: Assessment and Needs Capacity

- Area of Responsibility VI: Communication

Introduction

Health promotion and wellness have evolved dramatically since the earliest humans and are continually changing the way we advocate for health across the globe. The term "health promotion" has gained notoriety only within the past 30 years, creating a new innovative venue for health educators to advocate, enable, and mediate for health and wellness (World Health Organization, 2017c). Eventually, wellness gained currency throughout the early '50s to the late '70s, yet the origin of wellness had been around since ancient times (GWI, 2016). As health has grown and changed, we have come to see a new progression in the field that is leading towards health as not just a responsibility but also part of one's well-being (World Health Organization, 2017c).

Throughout this book, you will notice that at the beginning of each chapter (following the chapter objectives), there are links to the National Commission for Health Education Credentialing's seven areas of responsibilities. These areas of responsibility define the skills needed for entry-level health education and health promotion professionals. Each chapter guides professional preparation related to these responsibilities. The purpose of this book is to provide those who are new to the field a foundational background in health promotion and wellness through authentic learning, collaboration, practice, knowledge, reflection, and mobilization across the eight dimensions of wellness.

Within this chapter, you will find basic terminology and concepts that are crucial in understanding the foundation of health promotion and wellness. The progression of health promotion and wellness will be explained through several sections: (1) the development of health education, health promotion, and wellness; (2) the relationships among health education, health promotion, and wellness; (3) concepts and practice of health promotion; and (4) the ultimate goal of health promotion and wellness.

The Terminology of Health Education, Health Promotion, and Wellness

The terminology identified and defined in this chapter and used throughout the book is considered more common terms associated with health and health promotion. It is essential that readers gain an understanding of these key terms so they can build the foundation for the upcoming concepts and constructs described in this book. Just like the progression of health promotion and wellness, most definitions you will see in this chapter have evolved. As professionals in the field, we are always trying to use the most recent and useful terminology.

The definition of health has changed considerably over the years. We must first focus on the meaning of health as it lays the groundwork for all other terms identified in this chapter.

1. **Health**—"is a dynamic state or condition that is multidimensional (i.e., physical, emotional, social, intellectual, spiritual, and occupational), a resource for living, and results from a person's interactions with and adaptation to the environment" (Joint Committee on Health Education Terminology, 2012a, p. 10).

2. **Public Health**—"the science of protecting and improving the health of families and communities through the promotion of healthy lifestyles, research for disease and injury prevention and detection and control of infectious diseases" (Centers for Disease Control, 2017; e.g., all individuals, local neighborhoods, the entire country).

3. **Community Health**—"is a multi-sector and multi-disciplinary collaborative enterprise that uses public health, evidence-based strategies, and other approaches to engage and work with communities in a culturally appropriate manner to optimize the health and quality of life of all persons" (Goodman, Bunnell, & Posner, 2014). It is an aspect of public health that is focused on the health of a given group of individuals that is defined by locality (biologic community; e.g., college campus, workplace, neighborhood, etc.).

4. **Population Health**—"the health outcomes of a group of individuals, including the distribution of such outcomes within the group ... the field of population health includes health outcomes, patterns of health determinants, and policies and interventions that link these two" (Kindig & Stoddart, 2003). Population health is focused on the health of a given group of individuals that is defined by a specific characteristic. These individuals are not organized by locality (e.g., diabetics, African Americans, pregnant women, obese children, college students, etc.).

5. **Global Health**—is considered "collaborative trans-national research and action for promoting health for all" (Beaglehole & Bonita, 2010).

6. **Health Education**—"any combination of learning experiences designed to help individuals and communities improve their health by increasing their knowledge or influencing their attitudes" (World Health Organization, 2017b; e.g., community health seminar, college health course, high school health class, elementary health lesson, etc.).

7. **Health Promotion**—"enables people to increase control over their health. It covers a wide range of social and environmental interventions that are designed to benefit and protect individual people's health and quality of life by addressing and preventing the root causes of ill health, not just focusing on treatment and cure" (World Health Organization, 2016; e.g., good hygiene through interactive forums for children, laws/policies for smoke-free campuses/restaurants, awareness of risk through DWI demonstrations).

8. **Coordinated School Health Programs**—"an organized set of policies, procedures, and activities designed to protect, promote, and improve the health and well-being of pre-K through 12 students and staff, thus improving a student's ability to learn. It includes, but is not limited to, comprehensive school health education; school health services; a healthy school environment; school counseling; psychological and social services; physical

education; school nutrition services; family and community involvement in school health; and school-site health promotion for staff" (Joint Committee, 2012b, p. 16; e.g., school policies on tobacco use, K-12 health curriculum, "No Bullying" campaigns, "Stay Safe" after-prom committees, etc.).

The Development of Health Education, Health Promotion, and Wellness

Health Education

The terms "health education" and "health promotion" are often used interchangeably in the field of health, yet some distinct differences are important to comprehend (see **Figure 1.1**). Health education is made up of planned learning experiences that are connected to sound theories that help us explain or predict behavior and events. Aspects of health education and health promotion have been around since the earliest civilizations, whether it be through the creation of bathrooms, drains, or covered sewers. It has been handed down from generation to generation. It wasn't until the end of the 19th century that health education was starting to increase within medical schools (e.g., nursing; Cottrell, Girvan & McKenzie, 2013), and it was not until much later that health promotion gained recognition.

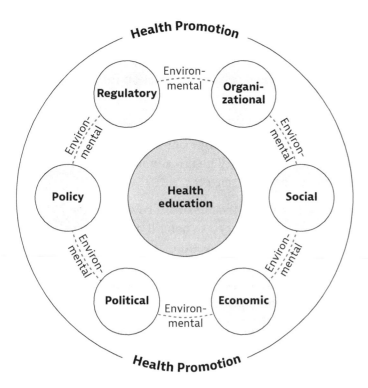

Health Promotion

Health promotion is the "promoting action taken by using educational, political, environmental, regulatory, or organizational techniques to maintain the quality of life within individuals and communities" (Joint Committee, 2012c, p. 101). The term "health promotion" was used for the first time in the mid-1970s (Lalonde Report, 1974). In the late 1970s, it was perceived as a form of health education that helped in influencing healthy lifestyles within individuals and communities (Davies, 2013). In the 1980s, the term was then broadened to incorporate individual behavior and the use of empowerment and advocacy to help improve the quality of life within individuals and communities (Davies, 2013).

Figure 1.1 *Health Education as the Nucleus of Health Promotion.*

Relationship Between Health Education and Health Promotion

Both health education and health promotion are considered eclectic because we pull concepts from a variety of different disciplines, such as biology, behavioral sciences, sociology, psychology, and many other health-related sciences (Cleary & Neiger, 1998, p. 11). It wasn't until October 27, 1997, that the Standard Occupational Classification (SOC) Policy Review Committee approved the occupation of "health educator." Today, health education and health promotion are considered to be an "emerging profession." Health education and health promotion is considered an "emerging profession" because we are unique in the sense that there is no required certification or licensure to be a health educator. However, we will discuss in later chapters certifications that are available for health educators to become specialists. Over the past 30 years, it has contributed to more comprehensive public health efforts across the globe, slowly moving towards gaining the recognition it deserves (Cottrell et al., 2013; see **Figure 1.2**).

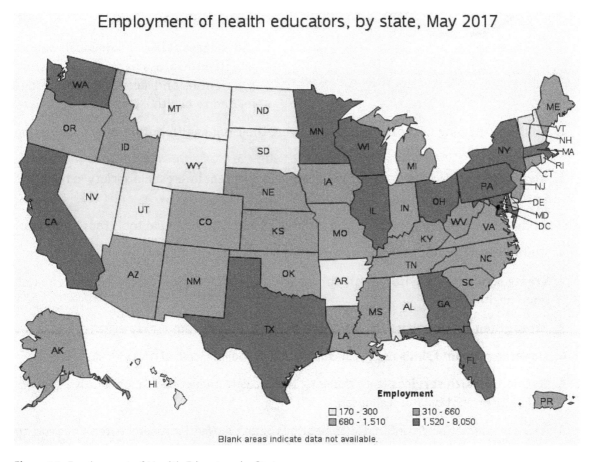

Figure 1.2 *Employment of Health Educators by State.*

Concepts and Practice of Health Promotion

The first International Conference on Health Promotion was held in Ottawa, Canada, in November 1986 and produced the widely recognized *Ottawa Charter for Health Promotion* (Nutbeam, 1998). The conference was held because of the growing public health movement taking place globally. This helped shape our understanding of health promotion and practical application strategies. The *Ottawa Charter* identifies three basic strategies for health promotion (World Health Organization, 2017c; see **Figure 1.3**).

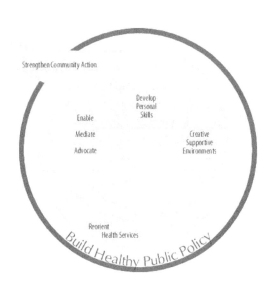

Figure 1.3 *Ottawa Charter for Health Promotion.*

1. **Advocacy**: public or individual support directed towards changing social, environmental, and economic conditions related to health

2. **Enabling**: helping all individuals in achieving their full health potential and increasing quality of life

3. **Mediating**: intervening or interceding between different interests in society in regard to health

The *Ottawa Charter* links these three basic strategies with five essential tools for promotion:

1. **Build healthy public policy** (e.g., accountability for health impact)

2. **Create supportive environments for health** (e.g., protection of factors that can threaten good health)

3. **Strengthen community action for health** (e.g., support community efforts)

4. **Develop personal skills** (e.g., philosophy, values, beliefs, self-efficacy)

5. **Reorient health services** (e.g., changing the focus from just clinical or curative services to health promotion and wellness)

The Fourth International Conference on Health Promotion (*New Players for a New Era: Leading Promotion Into the 21st Century*, which took place in Jakarta, Indonesia) expanded on the original strategies and tools identifying five significant priorities for the 21st century:

1. **Promote social responsibility for health** (e.g., actions of decision makers to pursue policies to promote health)

2. **Increase investments for health development** (e.g., optimize the health-promoting impact of public policies)

3. **Partnerships for health promotion** (e.g., work cooperatively towards shared health outcomes)

4. **Increase community capacity and empower the individual** (e.g., conceptual approach to behavior change)

5. **Secure infrastructure for health promotion** (e.g., resource mobilization)

These strategies are core elements of health promotion and are relevant for all countries (World Health Organization, 2017a).

As health educators, it is essential for us to understand and practice the basic concepts of health promotion. Health promotion is an essential element of one's health development and a critical investment (Nutbeam, 1998).

The Goals and Purpose of the Profession

The purpose of health promotion is the science and art of helping people discover optimal health, focusing on empowerment, advocacy, behavior change, and disease prevention. Optimal health is a balance of our eight wellness dimensions (physical, emotional, environmental, financial, intellectual, spiritual, social, and occupational health), and this will be discussed in the next chapter.

The ultimate goal of health promotion is to improve one's quality of life. As health educators, we would like to "increase the health expectancy and ultimately narrow the gap in health expectancy between countries and groups" (WHO, 1998).

Summary

In this introductory chapter, many basic concepts of the profession of health promotion were presented, including crucial terminology used within the profession (e.g., health, community health, global health, population health, health education, health promotion, wellness, and coordinated school health programs). The discussion of the progression of health promotion and wellness identified the starting point of the profession and the new innovative field of wellness. Then the relationships among health education, health promotion, and wellness were thoroughly explained so readers could identify both the similarities and differences of these terms. The basic underlying concepts of health promotion (e.g., advocacy, enabling, and mediating) were defined and explained through the *Ottawa Charter: The First International Health Promotion Conference*. Finally, a brief outline of the ultimate goal and purpose of health promotion and wellness was presented.

Review Questions

1. Explain the difference between health education and health promotion.

2. What was produced as a result of the First International Conference on Health Promotion? Explain what the three basic strategies were that identified health promotion at this conference.

3. Five necessary tools were then developed to take action on the above strategies. What are they? Provide an example for each.

4. Provide one example of each of the five major health promotion priorities for the 21st century.

Case Scenario

You are the new wellness educator for the American Heart Association, and your supervisor has asked you to work at a health promotion booth at a local women's health fair. While at the booth, you must utilize the three concepts and practices of health promotion to promote healthy living as a means of preventing heart disease. What will be your priority? Provide an action plan for how you will implement the three basic strategies for health promotion.

Critical Thinking Questions

1. Think about your school environment. Do you feel your college/university provides adequate health education to its students? In what ways?

2. If you were an attendee at the first International Conference on Health Promotion, what main health initiatives would you want the committee to discuss? What advocacy, enabling, and mediating strategies would you develop to help see your effort succeed?

Activities

1. **What does health promotion mean to you?** After reading Chapter 1, you have learned about the concepts and strategies of health promotion. Take a minute to compare your ideas of health promotion to what you have learned in Chapter 1. Do you notice any differences? Similarities?

2. **The First International Health Promotion Conference:** If you have not done so, locate and read a copy of the *Ottawa Charter for Health Promotion* created at the First International Conference on Health Promotion in November of 1986. It provides essential background information on the health promotion era globally.

3. **Through the Lens:** Chapter 1 has introduced specific content and standard terms used in the health profession. Through knowledge and reflection practice, identify these terms through a photographic lens.

    a. Assignment Steps

        i. You will be using your knowledge, reflection, and cultivating thinking to capture an appropriate image that relates to one of the critical terms described in Chapter 1 (e.g., health, health promotion, health education, wellness, etc.). You can use any piece of technology to take this image (camera, smartphone, etc.).

        ii. Once your image is captured, you must reflect on the meaning of your photographic image:

            1. How does this image relate to health?

            2. What term/concept is being represented?

            3. Define the term from the chapter information.

Web Links

http://www.who.int/healthpromotion/conferences/previous/ottawa/en/

The First International Health Promotion Conference: Ottawa Charter

This site introduces the progression to health promotion through all documentation of the First International Health Promotion Conference.

http://www.who.int/healthpromotion/conferences/previous/jakarta/declaration/en/

Jakarta Declaration on Leading Health Promotion Into the 21st Century

This site reveals the 4th International Health Promotion conference that focused on the new, improved priorities for the 21st century.

https://www.bls.gov/oes/current/oes211091.htm

Bureau of Labor Statistics – Health Educators

This site is rich in data linked to the employment status of health educators across the nation. The data shown gives readers an idea of the progression of health.

http://www.globalwellnessinstitute.org/

Global Wellness Institute

GWI is a nonprofit organization whose mission is to empower wellness worldwide by educating private and public sectors worldwide.

https://www.samhsa.gov/wellness-initiative/eight-dimensions-wellness

The Eight Dimensions of Wellness – SAMHSA

The Substance Abuse and Mental Health Services Administration (SAMHSA) is the agency within the U.S. Department of Health and Human Services that leads public health efforts to advance the behavioral health of the nation. This site goes into detail about the eight dimensions of wellness and their links to our everyday lives.

References

Beaglehole, R., & Bonita, R. (2010). What is global health? *Global Health Action, 3*(10), 1–2. doi:10.3402/gha.v3i0.5142

Centers for Disease Control and Prevention. (2017). *What is public health?* Retrieved from https://www.cdc-foundation.org/content/what-public-health

Cleary, M. J., & Neiger, B. L. (1998). *The certified health education specialist: A self-study guide for professional competency* (3rd ed.). Allentown, PA: The National Commission for Health Education Credentialing.

Cottrell, R. R., Girvan, J. T., & McKenzie, J. F. (2013). *Principles & foundations of health promotion and education.* New York, NY: Benjamin Cummings.

Davies, J. K. (2013). *Health promotion: A unique discipline?* Auckland, New Zealand: Health Promotion Forum of New Zealand.

Goodman, R. A., Bunnell, R., Posner, S. F. (2014). What is "community health"? Examining the meaning of an evolving field in public health. *Journal of Preventive Medicine, 67*(1), S58–S61. doi: http://dx.doi.org/10.1016/j.ypmed.2014.07.028

Global Wellness Institute. (2016). *The history of wellness.* Retrieved from https://www.globalwellnessinstitute.org/history-of-wellness/

Joint Committee on Health Education Terminology. (2012). Report of the 2011 Joint Committee on Health Education and Health Promotion Terminology. *American Journal of Health Education, 43*(2), 1–19.

Kindig, D., & Stoddart, G. (2003). What is population health? *American Journal of Public Health, 93*(3), 380–383. doi: 10.2105/AJPH.93.3.380

Lalonde, M. (1974). *A new perspective on the health of Canadians.* Ottawa, Ontario, Canada: Minister of Supply and Services.

Nutbeam, D. (1998). Health promotion glossary. *Health Promotion International, 13*(4), 349–364.

Substance Abuse and Mental Health Services Administration. (2016). *The eight dimensions of wellness.* Retrieved from https://www.samhsa.gov/wellness-initiative/eight-dimensions-wellness

The World Health Organization. (1947). *Constitution of the World Health Organization.* Retrieved from http://www.who.int/governance/eb/who_constitution_en.pdf

The World Health Organization. (1998). *The health promotion glossary online.* Retrieved from http://www.who.int/healthpromotion/about/HPG/en/

The World Health Organization. (2016). *Q&A: what is health promotion?* Retrieved from http://www.who.int/features/qa/health-promotion/en/

The World Health Organization. (2017a). *Jakarta declaration on leading health promotion into the 21st century.* Retrieved from http://www.who.int/healthpromotion/conferences/previous/jakarta/declaration/en/

The World Health Organization. (2017b). *Health topics: Health education.* Retrieved from http://www.who.int/topics/health_education/en/

The World Health Organization. (2017c). *The Ottawa charter for health promotion.* Retrieved from http://www.who.int/healthpromotion/conferences/previous/ottawa/en/

Credits

CHAPTER 2

The Eight Dimensions of Wellness

CHAPTER KEY

Authentic Learning: using problem-solving of real-life scenarios to explore and discuss content and concepts.

Knowledge: the theoretical or practical understanding of a concept.

Reflection: contemplation or meditation.

Practice: applications of ideas or concepts.

Collaboration: working with content from other organizations or peers.

Leadership: the act of leading a group or organization.

Chapter Objectives

After reading this chapter and answering the questions at the end, you will be able to:

- **Differentiate** among keywords, terms, and definitions related to the eight dimensions of wellness (*knowledge & reflection*).

- **Identify** the importance of each dimension to total wellness (*authentic learning, knowledge, reflection, practice, collaboration, and leadership*).

- **Describe** health and wellness as an integrated state of being (*knowledge & reflection*).

- **Integrate** the wellness dimensions into real-life scenarios and situations (*authentic learning, collaboration, and leadership*).

Chapter Links to the Areas of Responsibility of a Health Educator/Health Promotion Professional

- Area of Responsibility I: Assessment and Needs Capacity

- Area of Responsibility V: Advocacy

- Area of Responsibility VI: Communication

Introduction

The purpose of this chapter is to invite students into the world of wellness. To understand wellness, one must understand health. Health "is a dynamic state or condition that is multi-dimensional, a resource for living, and results from a person's interactions and adaptation to the environment" (Joint Committee, 2012, p. 10). Maintaining an optimal level of wellness is crucial for one's health and quality of life. Wellness is "an approach to health that focuses on balancing the many aspects, or dimensions, of a person's life through increasing the adoption of health-enhancing behaviors rather than attempting to minimize the conditions of illness" (Joint Committee, 2012, p. 10). One can reach **optimal wellness** by understanding how to maintain and incorporate each of the eight dimensions into their daily life. This chapter will consider each of the eight dimensions, their importance, and how to make healthy choices towards optimal wellness.

Wellness

The term "**wellness**" is comprised of eight dimensions: emotional, environmental, financial, intellectual, occupational, physical, social, and spiritual. Each of the eight dimensions needs to be balanced during your activities of daily living to be at your optimal health. The term "well-ness" has been applied and used in many ways over the years and is still continually evolving. The term "wellness" focuses on being in good mental and physical health.

Within this book, we will focus on wellness and the eight dimensions it incorporates, which were adopted by the Substance Abuse and Mental Health Services Administration (SAMHSA). This chapter will provide a more in-depth identification of these dimensions and their effect on health. The concept of wellness was first defined in 1947 by the World Health Organization (WHO, 1947). Tenets of wellness have been traced back to ancient civilizations (e.g., Rome & Asia), whose traditions have influenced today's modern wellness movement (Global Wellness Institute, 2016). Today more than half of global employers are using health promotion strategies, while a third of employers are using wellness programs within their companies (Global Wellness Institute, 2016). The chronic disease and obesity crisis have been raging worldwide in this century, leading to unsustainable healthcare costs, and a shift in focus to prevention and wellness from medical communities and the government (Global Wellness Institute, 2016).

The Illness-Wellness Continuum

Wellness is the full integration of all eight of the dimensions explained in this chapter and not just the absence of disease or illness. The **illness-wellness continuum** was created by physician John Travis in 1972, representing high-level wellness to the right and premature death to the left (Travis & Ryan, 2004; see **Figure 2.1**). This continuum shows that an individual moving more towards the right (high-level wellness) includes awareness, education, and growth. The move-ment to the left (premature death) includes signs of disease and disability. The illness-wellness continuum shows that medical treatment can treat disease, bringing an individual to a "neutral point" where there is no more prolonged disease or illness (Travis & Ryan, 2004). However, the

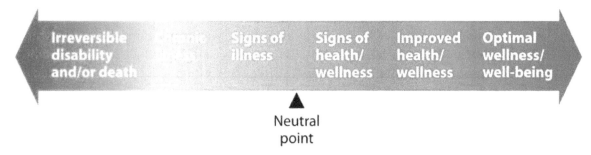

Figure 2.1 *The Wellness Continuum.*

absence of illness does not necessarily mean someone is of optimal wellness. One can have no signs of illness or disease but have problems in their mental or emotional dimensions. Wellness and one's well-being are dynamic processes, depending on where you are in your life, it is continually changing.

The Eight Dimensions of Wellness

This chapter will reference the Substance Abuse and Mental Health Services Administration's (SAMHSA) eight dimensions of wellness model (**Figure 2.2**). **The eight dimensions of wellness** consist of occupational, emotional, spiritual, environmental, financial, physical, social, and intellectual. Each dimension of wellness is interrelated with another and can affect each other, both negatively and positively.

Emotional Wellness

To achieve optimal wellness, we must start by evaluating our emotional wellness. **Emotional wellness** is a person's ability to cope with activities of daily living (ADLs) and create satisfying relationships (SAMHSA, 2016). This means inspiring self-care, being attentive to your thoughts and feelings, learning, and growing from experiences in a positive, optimistic, and constructive manner. Emotional wellness is essential because it allows one to express feelings and form healthy, supportive relationships with others. To obtain optimal emotional wellness, it requires positivity and a confident attitude that you can make healthy emotional choices. To stay balanced, there are a variety of strategies that can aid in your attainment of optimal emotional wellness:

- Smile
- Express gratitude
- Set priorities
- Cultivate awareness of feeling, emotions, and behaviors
- Accept mistakes and learn from them
- Seek support

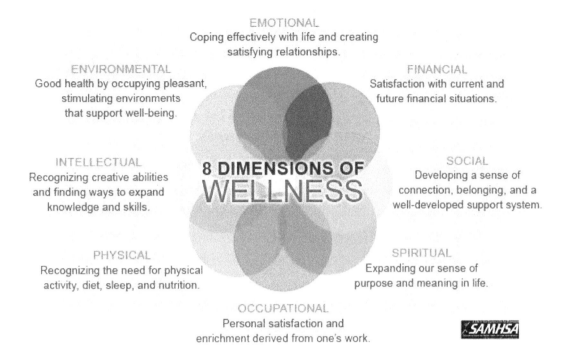

Figure 2.2 *Substance Abuse and Mental Health Services Administration's (SAMHSA) Eight Dimensions of Wellness Model.*

- Express emotions in a suitable manner

- Balance your other wellness dimensions

Evaluate your path to emotional wellness by asking yourself some simple questions: Am I able to maintain a balance of work, family, friends, and other obligations? Do I have ways to reduce stress in my life? Am I able to set priorities? Can I express my emotions in a positive, suitable manner? Do I balance all other dimensions of wellness? (A Strong Life, 2020). If you answered "no" to any of these questions, take a step back and think about the area for improvement, make it a priority, and set a goal for change. Emotional wellness is just one of the eight dimensions that require attention by an individual, and each dimension is essential in obtaining optimal wellness.

Environmental Wellness

Environmental wellness is another crucial dimension in obtaining optimal wellness. **Environmental wellness** consists of occupying pleasant and stimulating environments that support one's well-being and quality of life (SAMSHA, 2016). This means that one must be aware and respectful of their surroundings and lifestyle. Environmental wellness is practicing healthy habits that promote a healthy environment. By becoming more environmentally conscious, one can recognize how their habits may affect the environment. To obtain environmental wellness, it only takes a few easy steps:

- Become environmentally conscious
- Conserve energy
- Recycle
- Eat and buy local
- Volunteer with environmental organizations
- Be aware of natural resources
- Spend more time outdoors and less time with technology (phones, social media, television)

By achieving environmental wellness, we can all live in harmony and protect the world around us.

Financial Wellness

Another critical dimension is financial wellness, the process of learning how to manage daily expenses. When considering **financial wellness**, we evaluate the overall economic state of an individual. Good financial wellness will be determined if the individual is satisfied with their current and future financial situations (SAMHSA, 2016). More specifically, the individual is comfortable and thriving in their current living situation and can foresee themselves in this situation into the future based on a steady income. When either of these conditions is not met (dissatisfied with a current or future financial situation), one would be in poor financial wellness. To achieve optimal financial wellness, you can start with the following steps:

- Develop a budget
- Start a savings account
- Be aware of how you are spending your money
- Plan for major purchases
- Protect your credit
- Keep good financial records

Intellectual Wellness

Intellectual wellness refers to the knowledge and skill of an individual. When evaluating one's intellectual wellness, we must look at their creativity, problem-solving abilities, critical thinking skills, and motivation to expand knowledge. To enhance one's intellectual wellness, one can participate in creative and stimulating mental activities and share knowledge with others (NWI, 2017). According to Dr. Bill Hettler, cofounder of the National Wellness Institute, "It is better to stretch and challenge our minds with intellectual and creative pursuits than to become self-satisfied and unproductive" (NWI, 2017, p. 2). To achieve optimal intellectual wellness, you can start with the following steps:

- Find a good book to read for fun

- Engage in intellectual discussions or debates with your peers

- Learn a new skill such as a foreign language, play a new game, or learn to play an instrument

- Journal

- Use a planner to stay on task

- Engage in professional development opportunities

Physical Wellness

One of the most recognized areas of wellness is **physical wellness**. Individuals tend to be most familiar with the physical dimension of wellness because it is the most discussed in the media and the only visible dimension. Many think it is easy to identify good physical health; however, it is rarely seen as the multifaceted entity that it is.

Physical wellness is made up of nutrition, physical activity, and sleep (SAMHSA, 2016). Only when all three of these areas are adequately cared for can someone have good physical health and ultimately achieve optimal wellness. It is imperative to eat a well-balanced diet, participate in regular physical activity, and get the recommended amount of sleep. With that considered, physical wellness is highly debated. We know that diet, physical activity, and rest are essential, but what exactly should an individual's diet, physical activity, and sleep patterns look like to be at optimal physical wellness? Is everyone's the same? Who makes this decision? For example, physical activity consists of endurance, strength, and flexibility. How much of each is enough?

Other areas that must also be considered are drug and alcohol use, prevention through safety measures, and medical self-care (NWI, 2017). Even when the three major areas of physical wellness are in place (nutrition, physical activity, and sleep), drug and alcohol use, lack of safety precautions, and being uninformed about medical care can negatively impact physical wellness. To achieve optimal physical wellness, you can start with the following steps:

- Get the recommended 7–8 hours of sleep

- Get up and move every hour for at least 5 minutes

- Exercise at least 30 minutes most days of the week

- Eat healthy nutritious foods to fuel your body

- Stay hydrated

- Attend annual physical appointments with your doctor

- Avoid harmful teratogens such as alcohol, drugs, and smoking

Occupational Wellness

As with many of the other dimensions of wellness, **occupational wellness** is intrapersonal. It is one's satisfaction with the work they do (SAMHSA, 2016). Occupational wellness does not just mean having a well-paying job. An individual can have a well-paying job, but this does not mean they are fulfilled in their work. Good occupational wellness can be seen in those who use their job to help enrich their life. According to Hettler, "It is better to choose a career which is consistent with our values, interests, and beliefs than to select one that is unrewarding to us" (NWI, 2017, p. 1). Ultimately, both work and life should stimulate and inspire each other, and having a positive attitude towards the work one does can help enhance this symbiotic relationship. In addition to job satisfaction, professional choice, career ambitions, and personal performance should be considered to have good occupational wellness (NWI, 2017). To achieve optimal occupational wellness, you can start with the following steps:

- Stay motivated

- Get to know your coworkers

- Find a work-life balance

- Maintain time management skills

- Organize your workspace

- Take breaks when needed

- Set mini-goals for yourself

Social Wellness

Social wellness is both inter- and intrapersonal, and SAMHSA defines the intrapersonal aspects of social wellness as "developing a sense of connection, belonging, and a well-developed support system" (SAMHSA, 2016). There is a lot of emphasis placed on the individual and their sense of comfort. Alternatively, Hettler defines the interpersonal aspects of social wellness as making "willful choices to enhance personal relationships and important friendships and build a better living space and community" (NWI, 2017, p. 1). Here you see the emphasis is placed on the individual's interactions with the environment. Both the inter- and intrapersonal perspectives are equally critical in one's overall social wellness. To achieve optimal social wellness, you can start with the following steps:

- Practice self-disclosure

- Respect yourself and others around you

- Maintain a support system

- Laugh often

- Make an effort to talk to those who are supportive of your life daily

- Get to know your own needs so you can contribute to others

- Try not to criticize, judge, or blame others

Spiritual Wellness

Intrapersonal and interpersonal perspectives can also influence one's spiritual wellness. **Spiritual wellness** is "expanding a sense of purpose and meaning in life" (SAMHSA, 2016). Spiritual wellness is more than just religiosity: it involves the values and beliefs that provide a purpose in our lives. Some may have different views of what "spiritual" means. It could be factors including faith, values, ethics, and morals. Spiritual wellness is all based on one's own personal purpose and feelings. Spiritual wellness ultimately means one strives for harmony by working to balance inner needs with the rest of the world (National Wellness Institute, 2017). When you can find peace from experiences in your life, you are more apt to develop peace within your inner self. To achieve optimal spiritual wellness, you can start with the following steps:

- Explore your inner self

- Meditate

- Develop harmony

- Look for purpose in your life

- Practice relaxation

If you are looking to transcend into spiritual wellness, ask yourself these questions: Do you practice relaxation techniques daily? Do you make time for meditation? Have you thought about your purpose in life? Each of the eight dimensions is crucial in achieving optimal wellness and require strategic balancing to reach one's full potential.

Summary

It is essential to understand that each wellness dimension is connected. When looking at Figure 2.1, you see how each dimension is linked to the next. Think of wellness as a juggling act, and you have eight balls (social, spiritual, environmental, spiritual, physical, financial, mental, and intellectual) that you are trying to toss in the air at the same time continuously. If one ball drops, you throw off your balance, and most likely, the next ball will fall as well. This is the same idea when thinking about wellness. If our physical health is lacking—for instance, if we have the flu—it then affects our work (occupational and financial wellness) and our ability to go out and socialize (social health). It can continue to snowball to the other wellness dimensions. By fixing one wellness dimension immediately, you may be able to see an improvement in several different dimensions. However, if it takes us longer to pick up a ball, another dimension may continue to be negatively impacted.

Applying the eight dimensions of wellness in your lifestyle can lead to optimal living and a lifetime of wellness. The eight dimensions of wellness are used in a variety of fields, such as "health promotion and holistic health, and has seen a growth in 'helping professions' including coaching, counseling, and medical arts and practices" (National Wellness Institute, 2017). After reading this chapter, you should now be aware of the interconnectedness of each of the eight dimensions that contributes to healthy living and harmony.

Review Questions

1. Explain the difference between "health" and "wellness."

2. List the eight dimensions of wellness.

3. In your own words, define the eight dimensions of wellness.

4. Provide an example of each dimension of wellness.

Case Scenario

You are currently in your junior year of study at the local university, with a major in wellness management. You are shadowing the director of the county health department for your practicum experience to get a taste of what the job consists of. The county is the most obese county in the state and considered to be the poorest. You have been asked by the director to help in creating a new program that addresses occupational wellness in local businesses in the county. Her goal is to improve the overall wellness of employees and business owners in the county. What interventions would you suggest for a program that is based on occupational wellness? Knowing what you know about the county, what other dimensions may be affecting occupational wellness? How are those dimensions connected? Explain how you intend to plan and implement this occupational wellness program.

Critical Thinking Questions

1. Now that you have a thorough understanding of the dimensions of wellness, think about your own life. Do you feel you are healthy in all the dimensions? If so, give an example of how you are healthy in each dimension. If not, in what dimensions are you lacking? Discuss strategies you would utilize to make improvements to ensure you achieve overall wellness?

2. Reflect on the eight wellness dimensions and discuss which of the eight dimensions are considered both intrapersonal and interpersonal. What dimension should you work on intrapersonally? What dimension should you work on interpersonally? Explain why.

3. Look at the following dimension pairs and discuss how they impact each other both positively and negatively
   a. Physical/Financial
   b. Occupational/Mental
   c. Social/Intellectual

Activities

1. Create your wellness wheel by drawing a Venn diagram with all eight of the dimensions explained in this chapter. Bullet point key items that represent you in each of the wellness dimensions (e.g., physical wellness: exercise, normal checkups). Explain how each dimension impacts and is connected to the next. Explain what could happen if one dimension consisted of more negative health behaviors than another.

2. Do a web search to investigate what your county is doing to address all the dimensions of wellness within your community. Provide an example of how they are addressing each dimension. For instance, for economic health, do they provide easy access to healthy foods, or is the community considered a "food desert"? Also, indicate whether they lack in one or more areas. If they are lacking, what programs would you recommend they add?

Web Links

https://www.samhsa.gov/wellness-initiative/eight-dimensions-wellness

Substance Abuse and Mental Health Services Administration

This website shows how making each of the eight wellness dimensions a part of your daily life can improve health for those struggling with addiction and substance abuse.

https://www.mentalhealth.gov

U.S. Department of Health and Human Services

The U.S. Department of Health and Human Services is a great resource to aid in understanding emotional wellness and the different health issues that can arise on the illness-wellness continuum.

http://www.apa.org/helpcenter/wellness/

The American Psychological Association

The psychological help center explains various health indicators that are associated with emotional wellness. This website explains how health is impacted by emotional wellness and what some signs and symptoms are.

https://www.healthypeople.gov/2020/topics-objectives/topic/environmental-health

Office of Disease Prevention and Health Promotion

This government website provides a plethora of wellness information and leading health indicators for the nation. You can also use this website to find health disparities data for your activity questions.

https://health.gov

Office of Disease Prevention and Health Promotion

Another government website geared towards the health of communities and individuals. Significant physical wellness data and guidelines are represented on this website.

http://www.nationalwellness.org/

National Wellness Institute

The National Wellness Institute provides information from health promotion and wellness professionals in the field and provides extensive insight into the dimensions of wellness discussed in this chapter.

References

A Strong Life. (2020). *Environmental wellness*. Retrieved from https://astronglife.com/environmental-wellness/

Global Wellness Institute. (2016). *History of wellness*. Retrieved from https://globalwellnessinstitute.org/industry-research

Joint Committee on Health Education and Promotion Terminology. (2012). *Report of the 2011 joint committee on health education and promotion terminology*. Reston, VA: AAHE.

National Wellness Institute. (2017). *The six dimensions of wellness*. Retrieved from http://www.nationalwellness.org/?page=Six_Dimensions

Substance Abuse and Mental Health Services Administration. (2016). *The eight wellness dimensions*. Retrieved from https://www.samhsa.gov/wellness-initiative/eight-dimensions-wellness

Travis, J. W., & Ryan, R. S. (2004). *Wellness workbook: how to achieve enduring health and vitality*. Berkeley, CA: Celestial Arts.

World Health Organization (WHO). (1947). *Constitution of the World Health Organization*. Retrieved from http://apps.who.int/gb/bd/PDF/bd47/EN/constitution-en.pdf

Credits

CHAPTER 3

Historical Health and Its Influence on Wellness

CHAPTER KEY

Authentic Learning: **using problem-solving of real-life scenarios to explore and discuss content and concepts.**

Knowledge: **the theoretical or practical understanding of a concept.**

Reflection: **contemplation or meditation.**

Practice: **applications of ideas or concepts.**

Chapter Objectives

Upon completion of reading this chapter and answering the questions at the end, you should be able to do the following:

- **Discuss** health history from the earliest humans to the present day (*knowledge, reflection, and practice*).

- **Identify** community and public health initiatives globally (*knowledge, reflection, and practice*).

- **Identify** public health initiatives within the United States (*knowledge, reflection, and practice*).

- **Understand** and **apply** national health objectives through Healthy People 2020 (*knowledge, reflection, and practice*).

Chapter Links to the Areas of Responsibility of a Health Educator/Health Promotion Professional

- Area of Responsibility I: Assessment of Needs Capacity
- Area of Responsibility V: Advocacy
- Area of Responsibility VI: Communication
- Area of Responsibility VII: Leadership and Management

Introduction

Public Health

The term "**public health**" is a new term; however, the practices regarding public health have been in existence and continually changing since the beginning of civilization. As defined in Chapter 1, public health is "the science of protecting and improving the health of families and communities through the promotion of healthy lifestyles, research for disease and injury prevention, and detection and control of infectious diseases" (Centers for Disease Control, 2017a).

There has always been this idea of educating about health to improve quality of life, although visions of quality of life have changed drastically over time. This chapter will discuss health promotion through public health and how it has emerged in different civilizations worldwide. This chapter will go on to explore and examine the specifics of public health in the United States.

Evidence of Public Health in Early Cultures

There has been evidence of public and community health found in early civilizations such as India dating back 4,000 years ago. Archeological evidence shows that bathrooms, drains, and sewage systems as well as paved roads were evident in India (Rosen, 1958). Most notable are the oldest written health documents, such as the Smith Papyri, which dates back to 1600 B.C. (Rubinson & Alles, 1984). The **Smith Papyri** is a document that appears to be a textbook on surgery, starting with clinical cases related to head injuries (Breasted, 1922). The earliest written record of public health is known as the **Code of Hammurabi** (Cottrell et al., 2018). Hammurabi was the sixth king of Babylon, which today is an archaeological site in modern-day Iraq (Pearn, 2016). The code contained medical laws that pertained to health practices and physicians and the first known fee schedule (Rubinson & Alles, 1984).

Health Promotion and Wellness in Early Cultures

The Egyptians made significant progress in the area of public health, considering they are known as the cleanest and healthiest people of their time. Like the Indians, the Egyptians constructed sewage systems and drainage pipes (Pickett & Hanlon, 1990) and relied on priests for their health information. Like many other early civilizations, priest-physicians were used to help ward off evil spirits by using remedies such as body parts of animals (e.g., tissues and organs of crocodiles; Libby, 1992, p. 6).

In 1500 B.C., the Hebrews created what is known as the world's first written hygienic code, recorded in the biblical book of Leviticus (Oladepo, 1987). The law included personal and community responsibilities such as personal hygiene, protection against contagious diseases, isolation of lepers, disinfecting dwellings after illness, and specific hygiene rules for menstruating women and women who had recently delivered children (Oladepo, 1987).

In ancient Greek medicine, illness was viewed as a divine punishment, and healing of disease was a gift from the gods (Cartwright, 2018). *The Iliad* and *The Odyssey* texts provide information on how priesthood played a role in healing during this time. In *The Iliad*, **Asclepius** was a Thessalian chief who knew the use of drugs to heal, and he was viewed by ancient Greeks as the god of medicine (Libby, 1922). He had two daughters, Hygeia and Panacea, who also had healing powers. **Hygeia** was able to prevent disease, and **Panacea** could treat disease. Ultimately, Hygeia was more popular due to her ability to prevent illness (Libby, 1922). Greek medical practitioners began to move away from the connection of health and religion to more scientific inquiry. The Greek culture is said to be the first culture that put a specific emphasis on disease prevention and embraced the concept of balance among the physical, mental, and spiritual dimensions. One of the most famous doctors known, **Hippocrates**, the founder of the Hippocratic School of Medicine, made significant medical contributions that persist today. He developed the theory of disease causation and believed that health is the result of balance, whereas illness is the result of an imbalance among the wellness dimensions. The Hippocratic texts detail medical topics such as categories of diagnosis, biology, treatment, and medical advice for doctors (Cartwright, 2018). Hippocrates is also noted as the first epidemiologist (Duncan, 1988) because of his notations related to disease, illness, and geography during his time.

Eventually, the Roman Empire conquered the entire Mediterranean world, including the Greeks, creating their mark on history as well as in health. The Roman Empire (500 B.C.–500 A.D.) built an extensive and efficient water system that delivered an estimated 222 million gallons of water every 24 hours, and each Roman was provided with at least 40 gallons of fresh water per day (Rosen, 1958). They also created an extensive sewage system that was still part of the Roman culture in the 20th century because of how wide and high it was. Most notably, the Romans made significant health advancements, such as building the first hospital, acknowledging occupational health hazards, and creating private medical practices (Rosen, 1958).

Middle Ages (500–1500)

The Middle Ages, also known as the Dark Ages, was the era from the collapse of the Roman Empire to about 1500 A.D. Most of the health advancements, such as hospitals and medical practices, were lost during this time, and it was a time of social unrest. The Church replaced the Roman Empire and became the most powerful force in Europe. As the population grew, there was overcrowding, a lack of fresh water, significant problems with sewage removal, and a lack of personal hygiene and cleanliness (Rosen, 1958). The new religion of Christianity took over, and individuals viewed being virtuous as more critical for their next lives than sanitation and health in their current lives. As in some of the earlier civilizations, disease and illness were considered a sin. This brought priests back into the role of priest-physician, where they were again preventing and treating conditions. Many major epidemics occurred during the Middle Ages. The most inhuman and cruel outbreak was leprosy. **Leprosy** is an infectious disease that is caused by slow-growing bacteria in the nerves, skin, eyes, and lining of the nose (nasal mucosa; Centers for Disease Control and Prevention, 2017b). Because leprosy is highly contagious, individuals were forced out of their cities and required to wear bells around their necks to ring as warnings, wear identifying clothing, and wear rods that would identify them as lepers (Goerke & Stebbins, 1968). This isolation caused death, hunger, and physical harm (Goerke & Stebbins, 1968).

The **bubonic plague**, also known as the Black Plague or Black Death, is known as the most severe epidemic the world has ever known, with 5,000 to 10,000 deaths in a single day (Donan, 1898, p. 94). Estimates vary, but Europe lost one-third of its entire population, with total deaths equaling 20 to 35 million (Goerke & Stebbins, 1968). Bodies were dumped into rivers and church-yards and left due to the Black Plague being highly contagious (Goerke & Stebbins, 1968). One out of every four people contracted the disease, and dwellings were set on fire to rid homes of the illness. Symptoms of the plague consisted of blood and pus seeping out of sores on the body, fever, chills, vomiting, diarrhea, and aches and pains (History, 2020). The plague attacked the lymphatic system, causing a swelling of the lymph nodes and reaching the blood and the lungs (History, 2020).

The Middle Ages also saw epidemics, including **smallpox**, diphtheria, measles, influenza, and tuberculosis. The last significant epidemic disease of this period was syphilis, which appeared in 1492. As with other epidemics, syphilis killed thousands of people (McKenzie & Pinger, 2015).

Renaissance (1500–1700)

The Renaissance period was known as the "rebirth" period from 1500 to 1700. Science was again able to emerge, and many advancements were made; however, disease and the plague still lingered over Europe, and proper medical care was still hard to come by. **Bloodletting** was used during the Renaissance period and was a form of treatment for diseases and illnesses. Bloodletting was the withdrawal of blood to make one healthy again and was often done by leeches or a physician. Surgeries and dentistry were usually done by those known as "barbers." **Barbers** had the sharpest tools and the best chairs for surgical practices, similar to the chairs we see barbers using today. Living conditions during this era were filthy: floors were made of clay, and waste was never removed. However, living conditions for royalty were a bit different: they had basic hygiene necessities, bathed more frequently, and wore silk and velvet clothing (Hansen, 1980).

Scientific advancements and the exploration of the human body happened during the Renaissance era. John Hunter was known as the father of modern surgery, and Antonie van Leeuwenhoek discovered the microscope, proving that there were life forms too small for the human eye to see (Goerke & Stebbins, 1968). Health boards were instituted to help combat the plague, and by the 16th century, the health boards expanded their areas of control and jurisdiction over a variety of different systems. These included "the marketing of meat, fish, shellfish, game, fruit, grain, sausages, oil, wine, and water; the sewage system; the activity of the hospitals; beggars and prostitutes; burials, cemeteries, and pest-houses; the professional activity of physicians, surgeons, and apothecaries; the preparation and sale of drugs; the activity of hostelries and the Jewish community" (Cipolla, 1976, p. 32).

Age of Enlightenment (1700–1800)

The Age of Enlightenment was a period of industrialization and growth. The **Miasmas theory** was created, which stated the vapors or "miasmas" from rotting bodies or contagion could travel in the air great distances and be inhaled and cause disease in others (Duncan, 1988).

During this time period, Dr. James Lind, a Royal Navy surgeon, discovered how scurvy could be controlled through consuming lime juice. Often sailors who were on long sea voyages would acquire scurvy and be called "limeys." **Scurvy** is a deficiency caused by a lack of vitamin C. Edward Jenner discovered a vaccine for smallpox. In 18th-century Europe, 400,000 people died annually of smallpox, and one-third of the survivors went blind (Barquet & Domingo, 1997). Most individuals were left with disfiguring scars, leading to the nickname "the speckled monster" (Barquet & Domingo, 1997).

The 1800s

Health in the 1800s was at a standstill, with little improvement regarding public health. Due to overcrowding and new industrialization, the streets of London were filthy and full of both animal and human waste, causing disease and illness to be at high endemic levels. Diseases such as smallpox, tuberculosis, typhoid, and cholera were prevalent where individuals lived and worked.

Cholera is an infectious disease that became a major threat to the health of individuals in the 1800s (Boston University School of Public Health, 2015). Cholera is an unpleasant and potentially fatal disease caused by the bacterium *vibrio cholera*. The symptoms of cholera consist of painful convulsions, violent vomiting, uncontrollable watery diarrhea, and dehydration (Dobson, 2013). If not treated, many die within a short time.

Large epidemics of cholera arose in Europe and America, killing thousands of people: some estimate 50,000 people died of the disease between 1848 and 1850 (Boston University School of Public Health). In 1849, Dr. John Snow, who studied epidemiological data, published the first account of his "waterborne theory." Dr. Snow used a "ghost map" to inspect the drinking habits of cholera victims. He found that most individuals who were getting sick were getting their drinking water from the Broad Street pump. Dr. Snow was able to pinpoint the cause of cholera as foul water coming from the Broad Street pump (see **Figure 3.1**). The pump was later removed, and the epidemic abated. In retrospect, Dr. Snow made several contributions to the development of epidemiology:

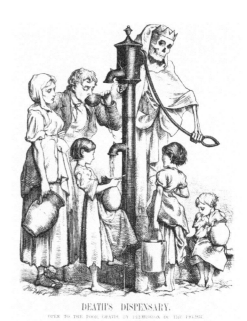

DEATH'S DISPENSARY.
OPEN TO THE POOR, GRATIS, BY PERMISSION OF THE PARISH.

- He proposed a new hypothesis for how cholera was transmitted.

- He tested this hypothesis systematically by making comparisons between groups of people.

- He provided evidence for an association between drinking from the Broad Street well and getting cholera.

Figure 3.1 *By removing the handle of the Broad Street pump, the epidemic was abated. The pump is still in place on Broad Street in London.*

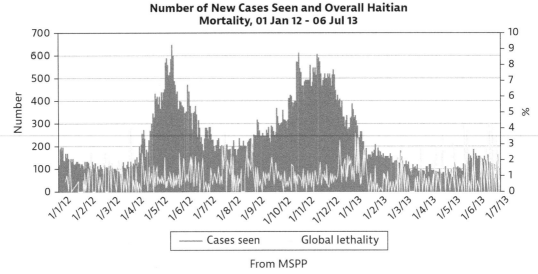

Figure 3.2 *Cholera Outbreak.*

- He argued for an intervention that prevented additional cases (removal of the pump handle; Boston University School of Public Health, 2015).

Cholera continues to be a problem today, particularly in the country of Haiti. An earthquake had devastated the country, where individuals were already struggling to find water and sanitation (Domonsoke, 2016). The disease struck with explosive force, infecting a new patient every 3 1/2 minutes in 2010.

In 1862, Louis Pasteur of France proposed the germ theory of disease. Louis Pasteur was a French chemist and microbiologist. The **germ theory** states that certain diseases and illnesses are caused by certain germs or infectious agents. Pasteur discovered how microorganisms reproduced, introduced the first scientific approach to immunization, and developed a technique to pasteurize milk (Cottrell et al., 2018). German scientist Robert Koch developed the criteria necessary to establish that a microbe, and no other, caused a disease (Cottrell et al., 2018). An English surgeon known as Joseph Lister developed the first antiseptic method for treating wounds by using carbolic acid, and he introduced the principle of asepsis to surgery (Cottrell et al., 2018). The second half of the 19th century (1875–1900) became known as the bacteriological period of public health (McKenzie & Pinger, 2015).

Public Health Efforts in the United States

The 1700s

During the 1700s in the United States, health conditions were like those of Europe, with human and animal waste causing illness and disease throughout communities. Diseases such as smallpox, cholera, and diphtheria were also present in the United States. Large numbers of immigrants were entering ports, and because of the slave trade, diseases such as yellow fever, yaws, and malaria were prevalent (Marr, 1982). In 1798, Congress passed the Act for the Relief of Sick and Disabled Seamen and enacted the formation of the U.S. Marine Hospital Services, which became the foundation of the Public Health Service (Boston University School of Public Health, 2015). Often seamen would become ill when out at sea and were unable to find health care when docked in port cities. Seamen were taxed 20 cents a month to pay the physicians, support the hospitals, and maintain their care at port cities (Boston University School of Public Health, 2015). In 1799, Boston, Massachusetts, established the first board of health and first department of health in the United States. At this time, Paul Revere was named the first health officer (Boston University, 2015). A measure of health status that is still used today is known as **life expectancy**. It is defined as "the average number of years a person from a specific cohort is projected to live from a given point in time" (McKenzie & Pinger, 2015, p. 608). The first life expectancy tables for the United States were created in 1789 by Dr. Edward Wigglesworth (Ravenel, 1970). Table 3.1 shows the expectation of life, according to Dr. Wigglesworth, in 1789. By 2020, the projected life expectancy at birth in the United States will be 79.5 years (U.S. National Center for Health Statistics, 2009).

The 1800s

Health conditions started to improve in the United States between 1800 and 1850. The Industrial Revolution was in full swing, and overcrowding, filth, and pollution were substantial in the United States. Disease and illness, such as smallpox, yellow fever, cholera,

Table 3.1 LIFE EXPECTANCY TABLE IN 1789

Expectation	Years	Expectation	Years
At birth	28.15	At age 50	21.16
At age 5	40.87	At age 55	18.35
At age 10	39.23	At age 60	15.43
At age 15	36.16	At age 65	12.43
At age 20	34.21	At age 70	10.06
At age 25	32.32	At age 75	7.83
At age 30	30.24	At age 80	5.85
At age 35	28.22	At age 85	4.57
At age 40	26.04	At age 90	3.73
At age 45	23.92	At age 95	1.62

Source: Ravenel, M. P. (Ed.). (1970). *A Half-Century of Public Health*. New York: Amo Press and *The New York Times*. Originally published in 1921 by the American Public Health Association.

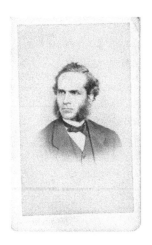

Figure 3.3 *Stephen Smith invited a group of gentlemen to discuss the possibility of a sanitary association.*

typhoid, and typhus, were still prevalent. Tuberculosis was rampant at alarming rates: in 1850, the tuberculosis death rate in Massachusetts was 300 per 100,000 people, and the infant mortality rate was about 200 per 1,000 live births (Cottrell et al., 2018). A major report, Lemuel Shattuck's **Report of the Sanitary Commission of Massachusetts 1850**, aided in public health reform in the United States. The report gave insight into how to approach and solve sanitary issues and public health in Massachusetts. The reason Shattuck's report is so influential is that there were no state or local health agencies at the time, and he visualized how to improve the public's health through the initial state and local health departments (Cottrell et al., 2018). As a result of Shattuck's report, full-time county health departments were created in Guilford, North Carolina, and Yakima County, Washington, in 1911. States started initiating boards of health where individuals would communicate and come together to problem-solve about the deplorable health conditions. From this, the American Public Health Association (APHA) was formed in 1872. Following a series of national conventions on quarantine held from 1857 through 1860, "Stephen Smith invited a group of gentlemen to discuss the possibility of a sanitary association" (Bernstein, 1972, p. 2; see **Figure 3.3**). Smith's suggestion interested community members, and an annual meeting was first held in Cincinnati, Ohio. Seventy members were elected at that time, and the APHA has been active ever since (Cottrell et al., 2018).

As previously reported, the Act for the Relief of Sick and Disabled Seamen, otherwise known as the **Marine Hospital Service Act**, was passed in 1798. This act "represented the first pre-paid medical and hospital insurance plan in the world, under the administrative supervision of what eventually became a public health agency" (Picket & Hanlon, 1990, p. 34). This idea of prepaid insurance plans was expanded on throughout the 19th century, when, in 1912, "Marine Hospital" was dropped from the name and retitled the U.S. Public Health Service. The mission of the U.S. Public Health Service Commissioned Corps is to protect, promote, and advance the health and health safety of our nation (U.S. Public Health Service, 2020). Today, the U.S. Public Health Service is overseen by the Surgeon General and is a diverse team of more than 6,500 highly qualified public health professionals (U.S. Public Health Service, 2020).

In 1879, Congress created the National Board of Health. The National Board of Health was created by an act "to prevent the introduction of infectious or contagious disease into the United States and to establish a National Board of Health" (U.S. Congress, 1879). The board was comprised of 11 members, seven of whom were appointed by the president; three medical officers from the Army, Navy, and Marine Hospital; and one representative from the office of the U.S. Attorney General (Michael, 2011). The National Board of Health was charged with "(*1*) obtaining information on all matters affecting public health; (*2*) advising governmental departments, the Commissioners of the District of Columbia (D.C.), and the executives of several states on all questions submitted by them—or whenever in the opinion of the NBH such advice may tend to the preservation and improvement of public health; and (*3*) with the assistance of the Academy of Science, reporting to Congress on a plan for a national public health organization, with special attention given to quarantine and especially regulations to be established among the states, as well as a national quarantine system" (National Board of Health, 1883). The National Board of Health stopped all operations in 1883, ultimately due to the foundation of the APHA.

The 1900s

The period from 1900 to 1920 is known as the reform phase of public health (McKenzie & Pinger, 2015). During this time, a lot of expansion was happening in urban areas, with many individuals still living and working in deplorable health conditions. New federal regulations were passed to maintain the health and safety of individuals while at work, known as workers' compensation laws. By the end of the 1920s, the movement for a healthier workplace was well established, and the average life expectancy had increased to 59.7 years (Cottrell et al., 2018). During this time, voluntary health agencies were forming to address specific health problems or conditions. For example, the National Association for the Study and Prevention of Tuberculosis was formed in 1902, and in 1913, the American Cancer Society was founded. Today, voluntary health agencies still play a crucial role in the prevention of disease and research advances in the field.

From 1930 through World War II, the role the federal government played in social programs expanded drastically. Prior to the Great Depression, medical services were self-funded (Cottrell et al., 2018). Throughout the Great Depression, self-funding could not meet the demands of those requiring aid. In 1933, President Franklin D. Roosevelt created numerous agencies and programs as part of his New Deal (Cottrell et al., 2018). Much of the money from the New Deal was used in creating hospitals, public health and prevention, control of malaria, and the construction of municipal water and sewage systems (Cottrell et al., 2018). The Social Security Act of 1935 was the beginning of the federal government's involvement with social issues and health. Funding was made available through the Social Security Act to support health departments and their programs and to develop sanitary facilities to improve maternal and child health (Cottrell et al., 2018).

Around this time, two major agencies were formed. The Hygienic Laboratory of the National Institutes of Health was created to learn the cause, prevention, and help cure diseases (U.S. Department of Health, Education, and Welfare, 1976). Today, the National Institutes of Health is the premier medical research center in the world. In 1946, the Communicable Disease Center was created in Atlanta, Georgia, and is now called the Centers for Disease Control and Prevention. The CDC is the world's leading epidemiological center and is a major training facility for health communications and educational methods (Pickett & Hanlon, 1990). The CDC's vision for the 21st century is "health protection, health equity" and a mission of "collaborating to create the expertise, information, and tools that people and communities need to protect their health through health promotion, prevention of disease, injury and disability, and preparedness for new health threats" (CDC, 2016).

In 1965, the federal government passed major legislation to improve the health of the United States population by enacting Medicare and Medicaid bills. **Medicare** was created to assist in the payment of medical bills for the elderly. **Medicaid** was created to assist in the payment of medical bills for the poor or those of low socioeconomic status. These bills have since provided

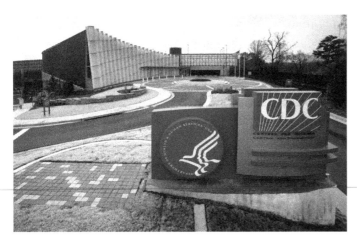

Figure 3.4 A general view of the Centers for Disease Control and Prevention (CDC) headquarters in Atlanta, Georgia.

millions of Americans with medical care that they otherwise would not have obtained.

The United States government continued to recognize the importance of health and well-being within the nation. A government publication titled **Healthy People** was first published in 1979, emphasizing that we move from a traditional medical model towards prevention by using lifestyle and environmental strategies. In 1980, *Promoting Health/ Preventing Disease: Objectives for the Nation* was published containing 226 objectives for the United States, divided into three categories of preventive services, health protection, and health promotion. These objectives and categories were used as a measuring tool to see where the nation needs improvement while providing baseline data (U.S. Department of Health and Human Services, 1980). These objectives led to publications being released every decade with the new objectives and baseline data for the United States. In 1990, *Healthy People 2000: National Health Promotion and Disease Prevention Objectives* was released, and in 2000, *Healthy People 2010: Understanding and Improving Health* was released. In 2010, *Healthy People 2020* was released, and we are now currently preparing for 2020 and the release of *Healthy People 2030*.

Healthy People 2020 is a guide for U.S. public health professionals and health education specialists for the next 10 years. There are 42 different topic areas that are addressed in this report. Programs are developed to initiate and try and meet the established goals and objectives for that decade (see **Figure 3.5**). *Healthy People 2020*'s mission strives to:

1. Identify nationwide health improvement priorities

2. Increase public awareness and understanding of the determinants of health, disease, and disability and the opportunity for progress

3. Provide measurable objectives and goals that are applicable at the national, state, and local levels

Top 10 Achievements in Public Health

1. Vaccination
2. Motor-vehicle safety
3. Safer workplaces
4. Control of infectious diseases
5. Decline in deaths from coronary heart disease and stroke
6. Safer and healthier foods
7. Healthier mothers and babies
8. Family planning
9. Fluoridation of drinking water
10. Recognition of tobacco use as a health hazard

Figure 3.5 *Top 10 Major Public Health Achievements.*

4. Engage multiple sectors to take actions to strengthen policies and improve practices that are driven by the best available evidence and knowledge

5. Identify research, evaluation, and data collection needs (U.S. Department of Health and Human Services, 2018b)

Local and state health departments and officials are encouraged to use these objectives and performance standards. Overall, the performance of public health departments and the health of Americans can be improved.

Table 3.2 HEALTHY PEOPLE 2020 TOPIC AREAS

1. Access to health services

2. Adolescent health

3. Arthritis, osteoporosis, and chronic back conditions

4. Blood disorders and blood safety

5. Cancer

6. Chronic kidney disease

7. Dementias, including Alzheimer's disease

8. Diabetes

9. Disability and health

10. Early and middle childhood

11. Educational and community-based programs

12. Environmental health

13. Family planning

14. Food safety

15. Genomics

16. Global health

17. Health communication and health information technology

18. Health-related quality of life and well-being

19. Healthcare-associated infections

20. Hearing and other sensory or communication disorders

(Continued)

Table 3.2 HEALTHY PEOPLE 2020 TOPIC AREAS (*CONTINUED*)

21. Heart disease and stroke

22. HIV

23. Immunization and infectious diseases

24. Injury and violence prevention

25. Lesbian, gay, bisexual, and transgender health

26. Maternal, infant, and child health

27. Medical product safety

28. Mental health and mental disorders

29. Nutrition and weight status

30. Occupational safety and health

31. Older adults

32. Oral health

33. Physical activity

34. Preparedness

35. Public health infrastructure

36. Respiratory diseases

37. Sexually transmitted diseases

38. Sleep health

39. Social determinants of health

40. Substance abuse

41. Tobacco use

42. Vision

Source: U.S. Department of Health and Human Services. (2018a). *2020 Topics and Objectives—Objectives A–Z*. Retrieved from https://www.healthypeople.gov/2020/topics-objectives

The 2000s to Present

In addition to *Healthy People 2020* and the upcoming *Healthy People 2030*, another great achievement was enacted in 2010. The Patient Protection and Affordable Care Act was signed into law on March 23, 2010, by President Barack Obama. This act is also known as the **Affordable Care Act** and Obamacare. Ultimately, this health care expands coverage to 31 million uninsured Americans and focuses on both prevention and prevention services (Open Congress, 2010). This bill will provide better access and affordability for those who were unable to be insured. It encourages and promotes worksite wellness programs, community-based prevention, wellness programs, and strong support for school-based health centers (Open Congress, 2010). Currently, in 2018, with President Donald Trump in office, there has been much debate about whether we should keep Obamacare. Today, in 2020, Obamacare is still enrolling citizens, but money and programs are continuously being chipped away at.

In November 2019, a large set of illnesses, including the common cold and respiratory infections known as coronavirus, appeared in the city of Wuhan, China. Currently, the illness is being called **coronavirus disease 2019, or COVID-19**. The COVID-19 pandemic is the defining global health crisis of our time and is the greatest challenge and public health emergency we have faced since World War II (United Nations Development Program, 2020). Since its emergence in China, the virus has spread to every continent except Antarctica, and the death toll is rising daily in Africa, the Americas, and Europe (United Nations Development Program, 2020). This pandemic and virus are devasting communities, creating economic, social, and political unrest that will leave deep scars globally. Students are forced to have schooling at home, parents have lost jobs, and there are mandatory stay-at-home orders for most of the country. The International Labour Organization estimates that 25 million jobs will be lost due to COVID-19 (United Nations Development Program, 2020). A mass shortage of face masks, protective equipment, ventilators, and COVID-19 tests plagues the United States. As of April 14, 2020, there were 1,956,077 cases of COVID-19 worldwide and 125,123 deaths (United Nations Development Program, 2020). This number is rapidly increasing and changing day by day and will continue to grow. Similar to people in the Middle Ages, we are engulfed in a pandemic that is rapidly spreading globally in 2020.

A Recognized Profession

One of the most historical events for health education and health promotion occurred on October 27, 1997, when the Standard Occupational Classification (SOC) Policy Review Committee approved the classification of the Health Educator (Auld, 1997). Health educators have been part of an emerging profession for over 25 years and were finally included as their own category in 1997. From this chapter, we can see that health has been around even before human time, and it is saddening to think that health education had not been a recognized profession until the late '90s. In addition to health education being established as an occupation, there have been 10 great public health achievements that occurred in the United States from 1990–1999 (see Figure 3.5). Today, we do not have to imagine a life without these great achievements. We are lucky to have vaccinations, family planning, and safer workplaces, but from history, we know that this was not always the case.

Summary

Health history is an important part of being a health educator and working in the field. It is important to know and understand how we got where we are today so we can effectively serve populations. By understanding the past, you can become a better leader in the present regarding prevention and health communication. Our concept of health education and health promotion today is much different than that of the past. We went from the earliest humans using trial and error to individuals in ancient times searching for ways to remain free of disease and illness. At those times, civilizations did not have the knowledge to understand disease causation or medical treatment, and individuals only relied on priest-physicians and superstitions to keep them healthy. In early civilizations such as ancient Egypt, there was a need for sanitation. Both Greek and Roman culture relied on keeping the mind and body sound to stay healthy. Some noteworthy achievements were made during those civilizations, such as the first hospital, better disposal of waste, and the formation of aqueduct systems. During the Middle Ages, much of these improvements were erased, and death and disease were rampant. The Black Plague, one of the most horrific epidemics of all time, nearly wiped out all of European civilization. Religion was considered a new means of health care; science and knowledge were shunned. The Renaissance period was a rebirth when science and health care were advancing, yet conditions were still filthy, and disease was still inevitable. The Age of Enlightenment provided the Industrial Revolution and the use of technology. Unfortunately, pollution and overcrowding in cities caused more disease and death. The mid-1800s brought advancements in epidemiological studies, which in turn found where the bacteria that was causing cholera was residing. In the United States, the 1800s brought a period of legislation: local, state, and county health boards were created to help reform the health issues within communities and within the nation. In the early 1900s, new medical facilities and medical treatment had been enhanced. Medicare and Medicaid were established to help both the elderly and the poor with financial assistance and access to health care and proper treatment. National health objectives were formed through the Healthy People initiative and are still in place today to combat major public health issues within the United States.

We have made great progress as a nation and globally in the field of public health, prevention, and health promotion, but we still have a long way to go. There are still many Americans without health insurance, in need of health resources, or suffering from new chronic conditions such as obesity, heart disease, and cancer. Globally, there are still many countries that do not have basic sanitary necessities such as clean water and sewage removal and are suffering from malnutrition and infectious diseases. As a health educator, you now play a critical role in educating populations about prevention and health promotion behaviors. By investigating previous health status in both the United States and globally, you are now better prepared to understand where we are headed in the future of health promotion and wellness.

Review Questions

1. Which cultures were considered the healthiest during the "early cultures"?

2. Explain the link between *The Iliad* and *The Odyssey* and their association with early medicine. What roles did Hygeia and Panacea play?

3. Explain the medical health advancements that the Romans made.

4. Explain Healthy People 2030. What are the objectives associated with this plan?

5. How has the Affordable Care Act impacted our health care system?

Case Study Scenario

As part of your job as a public health educator, you are required to investigate the impact that obesity has on your county. Your supervisor wants you to propose a prevention plan to the county legislators that incorporates the new Healthy People 2030 objectives. As part of the plan, you must present the H.P. 2030 objectives that you feel most adequately address obesity through an infographic or brochure for the legislators. During your research, you find that obesity is not the major public health concern for your county. How do you address this with your boss? Do you continue with your plan and infographic, or do you go against your boss and create a plan that targets the major public health concern for your county and present it to the legislators? How would you go about this scenario, and what would your final plan look like?

Critical Thinking Questions

1. Based on what you have learned about the history of health promotion, which time period do you think had the greatest impact on our current health care system? Health Promotion? Explain.

2. The Affordable Care Act has impacted our government in good ways and bad. Address the pros and cons of "Obamacare" and indicate how, as a health educator, you might revise the act.

3. Compare and contrast the Black Plague and the Coronavirus (COVID-19). How have these two pandemics changed the world and how we look at preventive health care?

Activities

1. You will need to extend a professional invitation to someone you may know (preferably between 60–80 years of age) to participate in a health history interview. This can be someone related to you, an acquaintance, a friend, a coworker, etc. You want to ask

them about their experiences during the period when they grew up. You can use some of the example questions below.

   a. What is your most influential memory about the time period you grew up in (e.g., major war, health crisis, technology, presidents, etc.)?
   b. What kinds of health care did you receive as a young child?
   c. Were seat belts required in vehicles when you were an adolescent?
   d. Was tobacco recognized as a health hazard when you were a young child?
   e. Was obesity a huge concern during your adolescence? If not, what was the major health concern?
   f. In regard to access to health services, was there a place near your home you could go if you needed health information?
   g. Did you have access to basic sanitary necessities such as toilets, baths, showers, sinks, clean water, etc.?

2. After the interview, reflect on any connections you found in regard to your health history interview and what the textbook has described historically about health education and health promotion.

   a. What were the similarities? What were the differences?
   b. How have we advanced since the earliest humans?
   c. How have we declined since the earliest humans?

3. Research Healthy People 2020 by logging on to the main web page. Choose one objective from the Healthy People 2020 target list and identify the goal and overview of that objective. List three objectives with their baselines and targets. What interventions and resources have been used in trying to change the baseline of this health issue? What needs to be done in the future in combating this health issue that was not listed on the Healthy People 2020 page?

Web Links

http://www.cdc.gov/museum/timeline/index.html

Centers for Disease Control and Prevention

This website displays historical health information in a timeline format, starting from the CDC's founding year, 1946, and continuing to the present year.

http://www.healthypeople.gov/

Healthy People 2020

The home page for Healthy People 2020 lists the national goals and objectives for the nation regarding various behaviors.

https://www.history.com/topics/black-death

The History Channel

This website explains "Black Death" and how it devastated mankind. Several videos and facts are used to explain what Black Death was and how it was one of the worst outbreaks in history.

https://www.nih.gov/about-nih/who-we-are/history

National Institutes of Health, Office History

The National Institutes of Health (NIH) website provides a history of the organization and how the main highlights of what the organization does.

https://www.apha.org/about-apha

American Public Health Association

This website explains current topics and issues in the United States today. The website also addresses policies, advocacy, and professional development.

References

Ambrose Video Publishing. (1995). *The Black Death: 1347 AD.* [Film].

Auld, E. (Winter 1997/1998). Executive edge. *SOPHE News & Views, 24*(4), 4.

Barquet, N., & Domingo, P. (1997). Smallpox: The triumph over the most terrible of the ministers of death. *Ann Intern Med, 127*(8 Pt. 1):635–642.

Bernstein, N. R. (1972). *APHA: The first one hundred years.* Washington, DC: American Public Health Association.

Boston University School of Public Health. (2015). *A brief history of public health.* Office of Teaching & Digital Learning. Retrieved from http://sphweb.bumc.bu.edu/otlt/MPH-Modules/PH/PublicHealthHistory/publichealthhistory8.html

Breasted, J. H. (1922). *The Edwin Smith papyrus: An Egyptian medical treatise of the seventeenth century before Christ.* New York: New York Historical Society.

Cartwright, M. (2018). *Ancient Greek medicine.* Retrieved from https://www.ancient.eu/Greek_Medicine/

Centers for Disease Control and Prevention. (2017a). *What is public health?* Retrieved from https://www.cdc-foundation.org/content/what-public-health

Centers for Disease Control and Prevention. (2017b). *Hansen's Disease or Leprosy.* Retrieved from https://www.cdc.gov/leprosy/index.html

Centers for Disease Control and Prevention. (2016). *Vision, mission, core values, and pledge.* Retrieved from http://www.cdc.gov/media/subtopic/factsheet.htm

Cipolla, C. M. (1976). *Public health and the medical profession in the Renaissance.* Cambridge, England: Cambridge University Press.

Cottrell, R., Girvan, J., Seabert, D., Spear, C., & McKenzie, J. (2018). *Principles and foundations of health promotion and education.* New York: Pearson Inc.

Dobson, M. J. (2013). Disease: The extraordinary stories behind history's deadliest killers. New York, NY: Metro Books.

Domonoske, C. (2016, August 18). U.N. admits role in Haiti cholera outbreak that has killed thousands. Retrieved from https://www.npr.org/sections/thetwo-way/2016/08/18/490468640/u-n-admits-role-in-haiti-cholera-outbreak-that-has-killed-thousands

Donan, C. (1898). *The Dark Ages 476–918*. London: Rivingtons.

Duncan, D. (1988). *Epidemiology: Basis for disease prevention and health promotion*. New York: Macmillan.

Durant, W. (1961). *The Age of Reason begins: Vol. 7. The story of civilization*. New York: Simon and Schuster.

Goerke, L. S., & Stebbins, E. L. (1968). *Mustard's introduction to public health* (5th ed.). New York: Macmillan.

Gordon, B. (1959). *Medieval and Renaissance medicine*. New York: Philosophical Library.

Green, W. H., & Simons-Morton, B. G. (1990). *Introduction to health education*. Prospect Heights, IL: Waveland Press.

Hansen, M. (1980). *The royal facts of life*. Metuchen, NJ: The Scarecrow Press.

History. (2020). *The black death*. Retrieved from https://www.history.com/topics/middle-ages/black-death

Learning Objectives. (2018). Retrieved from http://sphweb.bumc.bu.edu/otlt/MPH-Modules/PH/PublicHealth-History/PublicHealthHistory_print.html

Libby, W. (1922). *The history of medicine in its salient features*. Boston: Houghton Mifflin.

Marr, J. (1982). Merchants of death: The role of the slave trade in the transmission of disease from Africa to the Americas. *Pharos, 45*(1), 31–35.

McKenzie, J. F., & Pinger, R. R. (2015). *An introduction to community & public health* (8th ed.). Burlington, MA: Jones and Bartlett Learning.

Michael, J. M. (2011). The National Board of Health: 1879–1883. *Public Health Reports, 126*(1), 123–129.

National Board of Health. (1883). Annual report of the National Board of Health. Washington: U.S. Government Printing.

Oladepo, O., & Sridhar, M. (1987). Traditional public health practices in Nigeria. *Journal of the Royal Society of Health, 107*(5), 181–182. doi:10.1177/146642408710700508

Open Congress. (2010). *H.R.3590 Patient Protection and Affordable Health Care Act: Open Congress summary*. Retrieved from http://www.opencongress.org/bill/111-h3590/show#

Pearn, J. (2016). Hammurabi's Code: A primary datum in the conjoined professions of medicine and law. *Medico-Legal Journal, 84*(3), 125–131. doi: 10.1177/0025817216646038

Pickett, G., & Hanlon, J. J. (1990). *Public health administration and practice* (9th ed.). St. Louis: Times Mirror/Mosby.

Ravenel, M. P. (Ed.). (1970). *A half century of public health*. New York: Arno Press & the *New York Times*.

Rosen, G. (1958). *A history of public health*. New York: M.D. Publications.

Rubinson, L., & Alles, W. F. (Eds.). (1984). *Health education: Foundations for the future*. St. Louis: Times Mirror/Mosby.

Schouten, J. (1967). *The rod and serpent of Asclepius*. Amsterdam: Elsevier.

United Nations Development Program. (2020). *COVID-19*. Retrieved from https://www.undp.org/content/undp/en/home/coronavirus.html

U.S. Congress. Reports of the actions of the 45th Congress, Sess. 3, Ch. 202. An Act to Prevent the Introduction of Infectious or Contagious Diseases into the United States and to Establish a National Board of Health, March 3, 1879.

U.S. Department of Health and Human Services. (1980). *Promoting health/preventing disease: Objectives for the nation*. Washington, DC: U.S. Government Printing Office.

U.S. Department of Health and Human Services. (2018a). 2020 Topics and Objectives – Objectives A–Z. Retrieved from https://www.healthypeople.gov/2020/topics-objectives

U.S. Department of Health and Human Services. (2018b). 2020 Mission and Vision Statements. Retrieved from https://www.healthypeople.gov/2020/About-Healthy-People

U.S. Department of Health, Education, and Welfare (USDHEW). (1976). *Health in America: 1776–1976.* (DHEW Publication No. HRA 76–616). Washington, DC: U.S. Government Printing Office.

U.S. Public Health Service (USPHS). (2020). *Commissioned corps of the U.S. Public Health Service: Mission and core values.* Retrieved from https://usphs.gov/aboutus/mission.aspx

U.S. National Center for Health Statistics, National Vital Statistics Reports (NVSR). (2009). *Deaths: Final data for 2006,* Vol. 57, No. 14, April 17, 2009.

Winslow, C.A. (1944). *The conquest of epidemic disease.* Princeton, NJ: Princeton University Press.

Ziegler, P. (1969). *The Black Death.* New York: Harper and Row.

Credits

Fig. 3.1: Source: https://datavizblog.com/2013/03/30/dataviz-history-the-ghost-map-the-broad-street-pump.

Fig. 3.2: Source: https://www.slideshare.net/TomMahin/the-haiti-cholera-outbreak.

Fig. 3.3: Source: http://www.medph.org/apha/stephen-smith.

Fig. 3.4: Source: https://commons.wikimedia.org/wiki/File:Tom_Harkin_Global_Communications_Center_PHIL_8876.tif.

Fig. 3.5: Source: http://wwwapp1.bumc.bu.edu/lphi/publichealthtraining/onlinecourses/orientationtolph/orientationtoLPH3.html.

CHAPTER 4

Investigation of Health Status

CHAPTER KEY

Authentic Learning: **using problem-solving of real-life scenarios to explore and discuss content and concepts.**

Knowledge: **the theoretical or practical understanding of a concept.**

Reflection: **contemplation or meditation.**

Practice: **applications of ideas or concepts.**

Collaboration: **working with content from other organizations or peers.**

Leadership: **the act of leading a group or organization.**

Chapter Objectives

Upon completion of this chapter and participating in the critical thinking questions at the end, you should be able to master the following:

- **Define** epidemiology (*knowledge and reflection*).

- **Explain** how to use and measure health and health status (*knowledge, reflection, practice, and collaboration*).

- **Describe** the importance and current status of the government's *Healthy People* initiative (*knowledge and reflection*).

- **Identify and apply** the level of the prevention strategies used by health educators (*authentic learning, knowledge, reflection, practice, collaboration, leadership*).

Chapter Links to the Areas of Responsibility of a Health Educator/Health Promotion Professional

- Area of Responsibility I: Assessment of Needs Capacity

- Area of Responsibility IV: Evaluation and Research

- Area of Responsibility V: Advocacy

- Area VI: Communication

- Area of Responsibility VII: Leadership and Management

Introduction

The purpose of this chapter is to investigate the health status of the nation. Furthermore, this chapter aids in understanding the basics of epidemiology. **Epidemiology** is a basic science of public health, an essential quantitative discipline that relies on statistics, probability, and sound research methods (CDC, 1990). This chapter will discuss the study of health in a population and community practice. Like the practice of medicine, the practice of epidemiology aids in proper diagnosis and helps prescribe the appropriate treatment for a patient. This chapter covers concepts related to infectious diseases and noncommunicable diseases through the chain of infection and the multicausation disease model. This chapter will also identify the different levels of prevention as well as the governmental initiative known as Healthy People.

Measuring Health Status

Measuring the health status of the target population or community is essential in determining rates of change, the effectiveness of services, and identifying the source of an outbreak. Surveys are the most commonly used tools to measure health status because they are generated to the health area being investigated. For example, when measuring the health status of type 2 diabetics, you would ask questions related to A1C levels, body mass index, and sugar intake. Generally, survey questions are quantitative. When the population that is investigated is small, such as an individual in a community center, the process can be simple. However, when working with large groups, such as statewide and nationwide initiatives, collecting data can be very tedious work due to geographic location, limited rate of return, incomplete surveys, identification of the target population, etc.

Health is easy to define. However, it is difficult to quantify the amount of health in a community, population, or even within an individual. Most measures of health are expressed through statistics based on a traditional health model of death, disease, and injury. The statistics used to gather this information are known as *epidemiological data.* This type of data is collected at national, state, and local levels to assist in the prevention or control of disease outbreaks. Epidemiology is the study of the distribution and determinants of health-related states and events, not just diseases in specified populations (CDC, 1990). The following sections will explain how health, or lack of health, are described and quantified.

Rates

Some of the most common measures of health status are referred to in rates. **Rates** are measures "of some event, disease, or condition, concerning a unit of population, along with a specific point in time" (National Center for Health Statistics [NCHS], 2015, p. 442). Rates allow for comparison among data to assess the degree of change or effectiveness of service. Rates are also used to gauge the incidence of illness if a population is growing and how long individuals are living (life expectancy). **Mortality** rates refer to "the number of deaths in a certain group of people in a certain period" (National Cancer Institute, 2018a, p. 1). Mortality is often referred to as the death rate. For example, death rates represent the number of deaths per 100,000 people in the specific population.

Rates can also be described in other forms, such as crude, specific, and adjusted. **Crude rates** are expressed for a total population, and accurate rates are shown for a subgroup, such as people with a particular disease. **Adjusted rates** are also expressed for the entire population but can be adjusted for certain characteristics such as age (age-specific; **Table 4.1**).

Table 4.1 MORTALITY RATE FORMULAS

Rate	Definition		Example (U.S. 2008)
Crude death rate =	$\dfrac{\text{Number of deaths (all causes)}}{\text{Estimated midyear population}}$	$\cdot\,100{,}000$	813.2/100,000
Age-specific death rate =	$\dfrac{\text{Number of deaths, 45 - 54}}{\text{Estimated midyear population, 45 - 54}}$	$\cdot\,100{,}000$	420.6/100,000
Cause-specific mortality rate =	$\dfrac{\text{Number of deaths (HIV)}}{\text{Estimated midyear population}}$	$\cdot\,100{,}000$	3.4/100,000

In addition to mortality rates, **morbidity** rates refer to "having a disease or a symptom of disease, or to the amount of disease within a population" (National Cancer Institute, 2018b, p. 1). The morbidity rate can be further investigated in epidemiological terms to address the magnitude of the disease occurrence. Generally, there is always some level of disease present in a given geographic location, and this is referred to as an **endemic** (CDC, 2012a). An example of an endemic would be influenza, or the flu, which is very common during the winter and spring months. While endemic rates are the expected level of disease in each area, an **epidemic** is an unnatural occurrence of a disease outbreak. An epidemic is when the level of disease rises suddenly and the number of expected cases is higher than what is considered normal for that area (CDC, 2012a). For example, there was an outbreak of poliomyelitis, or polio, in the United States in 1952, when 20,000 cases of polio with permanent paralysis were reported (CDC, 2018). More recently, there was a measles outbreak in the United States during January 2019, with 1,276 documented cases (CDC, 2019). In the case of an epidemic, the outbreak is generally contained in a specific geographic region. In the case of the measles, it was contained in 31 states (CDC, 2019). When the outbreak spreads beyond this geographic region, it is considered a **pandemic**. A pandemic is "an epidemic that has spread over several countries or continents, usually affecting a large number of people" (CDC, 2012b).

An example of a pandemic is the spread of the Zika virus in 2015. It began in Brazil and made its way throughout both North and South America. Additionally, it has been detected in the Caribbean region, including Puerto Rico (Ryan et al., 2017). As of August 2016, there have been 91,692 confirmed cases. However, it was expected that there were over 444,884 cases that went unreported (Pan American Health Organization, 2016). More recently, another example of a pandemic that spread beyond its geographical region is the Coronavirus (COVID-19). COVID-19 is said to have started in China and has now spread to 188

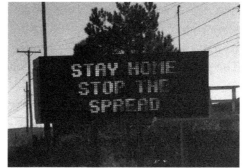
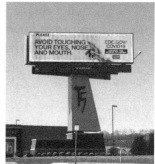
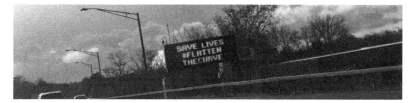

Figure 4.1 *COVID-19 Pandemic.*

countries and territories, resulting in more than 403,000 deaths and more than 7.03 million reported cases (Center for Systems and Engineering (CSSE) at Johns Hopkins University, 2020). Many countries restricted movement by issuing stay at home orders, closing borders, and stopping international travel putting countries in quarantine due to the deadly nature of the virus. Common symptoms include a fever, cough, and shortness of breath, recommended preventative measures include hand washing, wearing a face-mask in public settings, and maintain at least 6 feet of distance between other individuals. **Figure 4.1**, shows some of the strategies used within the United States to communicate prevention strategies in order to "flatten the curve" of COVID-19 and decrease the infection rates across the country.

Additionally, **life expectancy** is another means by which health and health status can be measured. However, it is also based on mortality. For instance, it is the average number of years of life remaining for a person at an age based on the mortality statistics for that time period. As of 2018, the life expectancy for a baby born in the United States was 78.7 years (CDC, 2017a). Regarding life expectancy, the United States ranks 53rd out of 100 countries, while Monaco is ranked number one, with an average life expectancy of 89.32 (Geoba, 2019).

Another means by which health status is measured is **years of potential life lost (YPLL)**. YPLL measures premature mortality and is calculated by subtracting a person's age at death from the current life expectancy for that year (CDC, 1991). This rate describes how prematurely an individual or group of individuals has died. In addition to calculating one's YPLL, there is a measure that specifically calculates one's burden of living with a disability (such as a stroke, paralysis, etc.). This measure is known as **disability-adjusted life years (DALYs)**. One DALY can be expressed as one lost year of "healthy" life or a life living without the disability (WHO, 2019). To calculate DALYs for a disease, you would calculate the sum of the years of life lost (YLL) due to permanent mortality in the population and the years lost due to disability (YLD) for the people living with the health condition or its consequences (DALY= YLL+YLD; WHO, 2019). This rate specifically refers to the **quality of life (QOL)** and, as health promotion specialists, we have to understand that just because someone is alive does not mean they are "living" their best possible life. The goal is to help individuals with morbidity concerns improve their QOL.

Leading Causes of Death

The overall mortality rates in the United States declined remarkably over the 20th century, resulting in large gains in life expectancy, but mortality rates from other causes, such as chronic diseases, have increased. Heart disease, cancer, diabetes, and suicide are now among the top 10 causes of death (see Figure 4.2).

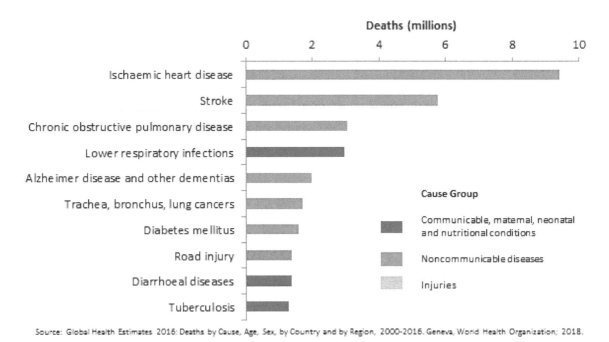

Source: Global Health Estimates 2016: Deaths by Cause, Age, Sex, by Country and by Region, 2000-2016. Geneva, World Health Organization; 2018.

Figure 4.2 *Top 10 leading Causes of Death Worldwide.*

Healthy People 2030

In order to improve health and eliminate mortality rates, the government initiative known as Healthy People was created. **Healthy People** is an initiative that was started in 1979 to improve health and wellness in all the Americas. It started as a government publication that first recognized the association of lifestyle to promoting wellness (U.S. Public Health Service, 1979). Healthy People is a 4-decade-old, 10-year national objective that focuses on the health outcomes in society. *Healthy People 2030* was released in December 2019 and is based on the initiatives from the previous years. *Healthy People 2030* is the fifth edition of *Healthy People*.

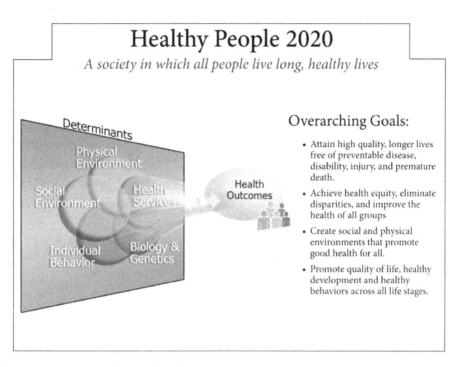

Figure 4.3 *Overarching Goals of Healthy People 2020.*

As depicted in **Figure 4.3**, there are many determinants of health, and each of these factors overlaps to some degree. It is imperative to recognize the association between the determinants when trying to improve the health outcomes. When referring to health outcomes, we must also be conscious of population disparities, such as race/ethnicity and socioeconomic status as well as gender, age, disability, sexual orientation, and geographic location (Healthy People 2020 Framework, 2010). Healthy People 2020 is composed of 42 topic areas, each with its own specific goals and objectives (Healthy People 2020, 2010). As of 2020, planning is underway for Healthy People 2030. The development of this initiative is a multiyear process that seeks input from members of the public, professional organizations, and diverse groups of subject matter experts (Healthy People, 2020).

The Levels of Prevention

Prevention, as it relates to health, is the planning for and the measures taken to forestall a disease as well as the occurrence of any other undesirable health event. When the term "public health" was first coined, there was a focus on treatment of disease with various sources, such as herbs, spirits, and natural remedies. Now public health focuses on the prevention of disease and health promotion rather than the diagnosis and treatment of diseases (CDC, 2017b). When referring to the term "**prevention**," the ultimate goal is to delay or stop an unfavorable event from occurring. In health promotion and wellness, this undesirable event is usually disease, illness, or injury. Prevention is categorized into three areas: primary, secondary, and tertiary (**Figure 4.4**). **Primary prevention** is intervening before health effects occur (CDC, 2017b; Canadian

Association of Physicians for the Environment, 2000). At the time of primary prevention, there is no current illness or injury. The goal is to reduce risk factors or risk behaviors for the disease/ illness/injury by reducing the risk of acquiring the pathogen or effect (Reisig & Wildner, 2008). Measures that represent primary prevention include vaccinations, positive behavior changes (such as increasing physical activity and wearing a helmet), and reducing consumption of substances that are associated with disease or illness. **Secondary prevention** is focused on reducing the prevalence or consequences related to disease and illness. During secondary prevention, there are no present symptoms but it is essential to identify and treat asymptomatic persons (Reisig & Wildner, 2008). Even though asymptomatic, a person may have developed risk factors that increase their likelihood of disease, and detecting it at this stage can delay or prevent the onset. This is crucial because early detection is key to prevention. Measures that can be taken during secondary prevention are screenings, tests, and regular checkups or exams. **Tertiary prevention** is managing the disease, illness, or injury post-diagnosis (CDC, 2017b; Canadian Association of Physicians for the Environment, 2000). The three aims of tertiary prevention are to (1) alleviate symptoms; (2) prevent subsequent disability; and (3) prevent the progression of the disease, illness, or injury (Grill, Reinhardt, & Stucki, 2008). Measures in tertiary prevention include rehabilitation programs, chronic disease management programs (e.g., for diabetes, arthritis, depression, etc.), support groups (allow members to share strategies for living well), and vocational rehabilitation programs (to retrain workers for new jobs) (Institute for Work & Health, 2006).

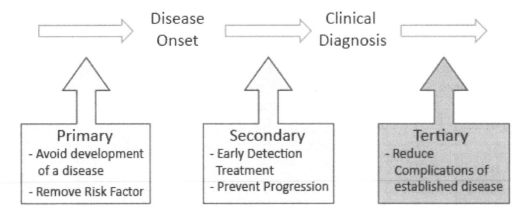

Figure 4.4 *The Three Levels of Prevention.*

Chain of Infection for Communicable Diseases

For one to prevent the onset of disease and illness, they must be aware of the chain of infection and communicable diseases. **Communicable diseases** are those caused by pathogens or disease agents and can be spread from one host to another. These hosts can include humans, non-humans, and animals. The American Public Health Association (APHA; 2018) lists more than 200 communicable diseases, including Zika, Ebola, Dengue, influenza, and Lyme Disease. **The chain of infection** is a model that represents the spread of communicable diseases from one host to another (**Figure 4.5**). Represented in the model are six chain links, each an agent in the transmission of infection from an infected host to an uninfected host. For this transmission of a communicable disease to take place, all six links must be present. A break in the chain will prevent transmission of the **pathogen** to the uninfected host. Strategies to break the chain at each of the links are listed in Figure 4.5. For example, the spread of HIV can be prevented at the portal of entry if a condom is worn by the infected host. With COIVD-19 the transmission chain can be broken if you avoid shaking hands or hugging to reduce transmission. Similarly, the flu can be prevented at the portal of exit if a mask is worn. It is important for health education specialists to understand how to break this chain at each link to be able to promote communicable disease prevention.

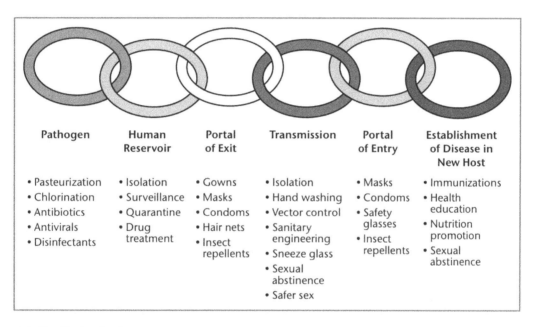

Figure 4.5 *The Chain of Infection.*

Multicausation Disease Model for Noncommunicable Diseases

Not all diseases are communicable, or pathogen caused. **Noncommunicable diseases**, or chronic disease, are those that exist in an individual for a long duration of time and progress slowly (WHO, 2013). Examples of noncommunicable diseases are cardiovascular disease (heart attack and stroke), respiratory disease (chronic obstructive pulmonary disease and asthma), and diabetes. The **multicausation disease model** identifies the five major risk factors for chronic disease (**Figure 4.6**). These risk factors, moving from intrinsic to extrinsic, include genetics, behavior

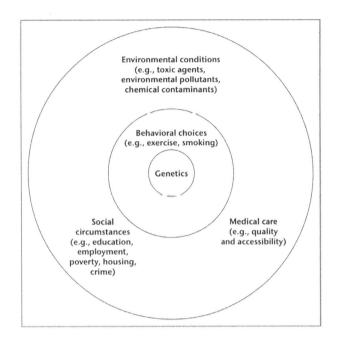

Figure 4.6 *Multicausation Disease Model.*

choices, medical care, social circumstances, and environmental conditions. Each of the risk factors weighs differently on the likelihood of chronic disease. For example, an individual who has a family history of stroke and currently smokes would increase their risk of cardiovascular disease due to genetics and behavior choices. The role of the health promotion specialist is to create programs that directly impact each of these risk factors to meet the needs of those they serve.

Summary

In this chapter, several concepts surrounding health data were presented, including definitions of many of the keywords and terms used in the profession: *mortality, morbidity, epidemic, endemic, pandemic, life expectancy, YPLL, DALY, Healthy People, levels of prevention, chain of infection, multicausation disease model, and communicable and noncommunicable diseases.* We included a brief discussion of the current status of health education and health promotion and a look into how health and health status has been measured. An explanation of the determinants of health, with a breakdown of the levels of prevention, risk factors, and understanding of disease, was outlined for the up-and-coming health professional.

Review Questions

1. Explain the differences among primary prevention, secondary prevention, and tertiary prevention.

2. Calculate the years of potential life lost (YPLL) if an individual passed away at the age of 36.

3. Explain how the chain of infection would progress with a bacterial disease such as MRSA.

4. Provide two overarching goals of Healthy People 2030.

Case Scenario

As a health education specialist at the local Oswego County Health Department, you have been tasked with presenting on HIV/AIDS at the local high school. However, you know that many parents in the community are against you coming in and discussing HIV/AIDS with their children because the topic is too controversial for the community. There is a fear amongst the parents that you will be promoting sexual activity. You have decided to create a PowerPoint presentation on HIV/AIDS that incorporates information on risk factors, chain of infection, and prevention methods. To make sure that you are on target with what the county is expecting for this presentation, you ask some of your colleagues for advice. Explain what you think your colleagues would brainstorm for you. What would they advise you to include? What would they advise you not to include, and why? Address what form of presentation they think would be most beneficial for this target population.

Critical Thinking Questions

1. Create a program for the community in which you live. What would be the target health issue you choose, and why? Make sure your program aligns with one of the three levels of prevention.

2. Looking at Figure 4.3 in this chapter, what Healthy People topic objectives are the most interesting to you, and what topic/health areas did you see missing from the table? Why do you think they are missing? Explain what topic areas should be of primary focus for Healthy People 2030.

3. There were 235 homicide deaths in Syracuse, New York, in 2011. The estimated mid-year population was 25,000 in 2011. How many homicide deaths per 100,000 of the population occurred in Syracuse in 2011? What type of rate is this? Solve this problem by providing formula and final calculation.

Activities

1. Partner with a fellow health education specialist and recreate the multicausation disease model to help explain how one develops diabetes. Be creative in your construction of the model (e.g., poster board, PowerPoint, etc.).

2. Research the Healthy People 2030 initiative and what the new topic areas and objectives are. How does Healthy People 2030 differ from 2020, 2010, 2000? Explain by writing a one-page paper.

3. Think about the past as well as the present and research one epidemic, one endemic, and one pandemic that has devasted the United States (refer back to Chapter 3: Historical Health and its Influence on Wellness). How have each impacted (1) you, (2) your family, and (3) your community? Create a PowerPoint presentation to present to your classmates.

Web Links

http://www.geoba.se/population.php?pc=world&type=15

The World Life Expectancy

This site provides an overview of 100 countries and their ranking of life expectancy. This gives students the ability to visualize where the United States ranks in relation to other countries.

https://www.healthypeople.gov/2020/topics-objectives

Healthy People 2020

This link provides an explanation of each of the topics and objective areas within Healthy People 2020. Each topic area includes an overview, objectives and data, and evidence-based resources.

https://www.healthypeople.gov/2020/About-Healthy-People/Development-Healthy-People-2030

Healthy People 2030

Planning is now underway for Healthy People 2030! Learn about the Healthy People initiative and how to get involved by visiting this website.

https://www.cdc.gov/nchs/index.htm

National Center for Health Statistics (NCHS)

This site is a gateway to a plethora of health data in the United States. NCHS provides statistical information that helps guides policies to improve the health of the American people.

https://www.who.int/healthinfo/global_burden_disease/metrics_daly/en/

WHO Metrics: Disability-Adjusted Life Year (DALYs)

An overview of health statistics and information systems that helps quantify the burden of disease from mortality and morbidity, including DALYs.

https://www.cdc.gov/hiv/basics/

HIV Basics

This link will help students address the case study scenario in this chapter. The CDC addresses basic information about HIV/AIDS and basic statistics.

References

American Public Health Association. (2018). *Control of communicable diseases*. Retrieved from https://www. apha.org/ccdm

Canadian Association of Physicians for the Environment. Primary prevention. (2000). *Children's environmental health project*. Retrieved from: http://www.cape.ca/children/prev.html

Centers for Disease Control and Prevention. (1990). *Principles of epidemiology: Self-study course 3030-G*. U.S. Dept. of Health and Human Services, Public Health Service, Centers for Disease Control and Prevention, Epidemiology Program Office, Division of Media, and Training Services. Atlanta, GA.

Centers for Disease Control and Prevention. (1991). Update: years of potential life lost before age 65—the United States, 1988 and 1989. *MMWR, 40*:60–2.

Centers for Disease Control and Prevention. (2012a). *Principles of epidemiology in public health practice* (3rd ed.). Retrieved from https://www.cdc.gov/ophss/csels/dsepd/ss1978/ss1978.pdf

Centers for Disease Control and Prevention. (2012b). *An introduction to applied epidemiology and biostatistics*. Retrieved from https://www.cdc.gov/ophss/csels/dsepd/ss1978/lesson1/section11.html

Centers for Disease Control and Prevention. (2017a). *Life expectancy*. Retrieved from https://www.cdc.gov/ nchs/fastats/life-expectancy.htm

Centers for Disease Control and Prevention. (2017b). *Picture of America*. Retrieved from https://www.cdc.gov/ pictureofamerica/pdfs/picture_of_america_prevention.pdf

Centers for Disease Control and Prevention. (2018). *Manual for the surveillance of vaccine-preventable diseases*. Retrieved from https://www.cdc.gov/ncird/index.html

Centers for Disease Control and Prevention (2019). Measles. Retrieved from https://www.cdc.gov/measles/ cases-outbreaks.html

Center for Systems and Engineering (CSSE) at Johns Hopkins University. (2020). *COVID-19 dashboard: ArcGIS*. Retrieved from https://gisanddata.maps.arcgis.com/apps/opsdashboard/index.html#/ bda7594740fd40299423467b48e9ecf6

Geoba.Se. (2019). *The world life expectancy, 2019*. Retrieved from http://www.geoba.se/population. php?pc=world&type=15

Grill, E., Reinhardt, J., & Stucki, G. (2008). Prevention, tertiary. In W. Kirch (Ed.), *Encyclopedia of Public Health*. Springer, Dordrecht. doi: https://doi.org/10.1007/978-1-4020-5614-7

Healthy People. (2020). *Development of the national health promotion and disease prevention objectives for 2030*. Retrieved from https://www.healthypeople.gov/2020/About-Healthy-People/ Development-Healthy-People-2030

Institute for Work & Health. (2015, April). Primary, secondary and tertiary prevention. Retrieved from https:// www.iwh.on.ca/what-researchers-mean-by/primary-secondary-and-tertiary-prevention

Minino, A.M., Xu, J., & Kochanek, K. D. (2010). Deaths: Preliminary data for 2008. *National Vital Statistics Reports, 59*(2), 1–72.

National Cancer Institute at the National Institutes of Health. (2018). *NCI dictionary of cancer terms*. Retrieved from https://www.cancer.gov/publications/dictionaries/cancer-terms/def/morbidity

National Center for Health Statistics (NCHS). (2015). *Health, United States, 2014: With special feature on adults aged 55–64*. Hyattsville, MD: National Center for Health Statistics.

Pan American Health Organization (PAHO). (2016). Zika virus infection. Retrieved from http://www.paho.org/ hq/index.php?option=com_content&view=article&id=11585&Itemid=41688&lang=en

Reisig, V., & Wildner, M. (2008). Prevention, primary. In W. Kirch (Ed.), *Encyclopedia of public health*. Dordrecht, NL: Springer. doi: https://doi.org/10.1007/978-1-4020-5614-7

Ryan, S. J., Carlson, C. J., Stewart-Ibarra, A. M., Borbor-Cordova, M. J., Romero, M. M., Cox, S., ... Ahmed, S. (2017). Outbreak of Zika virus infections, Dominica, 2016. *Emerging Infectious Diseases, 23*(11), 1926–1927. https://dx.doi.org/10.3201/eid2311.171140

U.S. Department of Health and Human Services, National Center for Health Statistics. (2010). *Health, United States, 2009: With special feature on medical technology.* Hyattsville, MD: Author.

U.S. Department of Health and Human Services. (2010). *Healthy people 2020 framework.* Retrieved from https://healthypeople.gov/sites/default/files/HP2020Framework.pdf

U.S. Public Health Service. (1979). *Healthy people: The surgeon general's report on health promotion and disease prevention.* Washington, DC: U.S. Government Printing Office.

World Health Organization (WHO). (2013). *10 facts on noncommunicable diseases.* Retrieved from http://www.who.int/features/factfiles/noncommunicable_diseases/en/

World Health Organization (WHO). (2019). *Metrics: Disability-adjusted life year (DALY).* Retrieved from https://www.who.int/healthinfo/global_burden_disease/metrics_daly/en/

Credits

CHAPTER 5

The New Role of Information Technology in Health and Wellness

Stephen Papay, ATC, LMT, CR-L1

CHAPTER KEY

Authentic Learning: **using problem-solving of real-life scenarios to explore and discuss content and concepts.**

Knowledge: **the theoretical or practical understanding of a concept.**

Reflection: **contemplation or meditation.**

Practice: **applications of ideas or concepts.**

Collaboration: **working with content from other organizations or peers.**

Leadership: **the act of leading a group or organization.**

Chapter Objectives

After reading this chapter and answering the questions at the end of this chapter, you will be able to:

- **Identify** the different areas in which we can find technology in health promotion and wellness (*authentic learning, knowledge, reflection, practice, collaboration, and leadership*).

- **Describe** how technology is/can be used in health promotion and wellness as well as other health-related fields (*knowledge & reflection*).

- **Integrate** the technology into real-life scenarios and situations (*authentic learning, collaboration, and leadership*).

Chapter Links to the Areas of Responsibility of a Health Educator/Health Promotion Professional

- Area of Responsibility I: Assessment of Needs Capacity

- Area of Responsibility V: Advocacy

- Area of Responsibility VI: Communication

- Area of Responsibility VII: Leadership and Management

- Area of Responsibility VIII: Ethics and Professionalism

Introduction

The purpose of this chapter is to introduce technology within health promotion and wellness and the healthcare field. The term "technology" refers to computers, cell phones, tablets, the Internet, email, and various other modalities. While you may consider this to be a new area within the field of health promotion and wellness, it dates back to the mid-1970s with computer-based teaching regarding venereal disease (VD; Van Cura, Jensen, Greist, Lewis, & Frey, 1975). Van Cura et al. required users to come to a location and use a computer to learn about VD. Fast-forward 43 years, and we're now using technologically advanced computers (smartphones, tablets, laptops) that give us immediate feedback on medical concerns (Stop, Breathe & Think, 2018).

With technology expanding so rapidly, it's very likely that what you are reading right now is outdated by at least 6 months, and devices that you use will have a newer edition available (Android/Apple products). Also, as technology begins to expand, the digital divide begins to decrease. **Digital divide** is a term used to describe a barrier between current technological trends and devices based on a person's socioeconomic status and geographic location. While it still exists to some extent, advancements in technology, the increased number of communication satellites orbiting the earth, and the affordability of new devices have helped decrease this divide. Due to this decrease, smartphones, tablets, laptops, and desktops can be found in many homes. With increased accessibility comes increased demand. People used to keep their phones for years before replacing them. Nowadays people will replace their current mobile devices with the newest models each time they are released. This quick turnover is also accurate regarding applications used by smartphone users. As you will read later in the chapter, specific applications for smartphones and tablets will no longer exist, and certain social media platforms will have faded away. Therefore, we must view technology as it relates to this area with a wide lens.

How Technology Shapes Us

As the world changes, new generations of learners emerge. Not all of these learners come from the same place, either. As with many aspects of life, depending on your cultural background, socioeconomic status, where you live, and age, you may do things differently or may have barriers to work around, such as transportation, access to resources, or even financial means. In the world of technology, these barriers are known as the digital divide (Bull, 2011). This divide often prevented specific populations from accessing new technology and current information. This digital divide has decreased over the years, though. This is due to the influx of affordable smartphones. However, the increased accessibility to these devices has led to an increase in usage, specifically Social Networking Site (SNS) usage (e.g., Facebook, Snapchat, Instagram). Many researchers are now looking into smartphone addiction in digital natives or individuals who have always had access to these devices/platforms.

Have you ever thought to yourself, "I couldn't survive a day without my phone"? In the case of Samaha and Hawi (2015), this is true for some people. Their researchers studied the correlation between smartphone use/addiction, stress, academic performance, and satisfaction with life. While this study did not find a relationship between smartphone addiction and satisfaction with life, it did find smartphone addiction has negative impacts on health (Figure 5.1 Samaha & Hawi, 2015).

This research, as well as the research of many other scholars, shows us smartphones alter the way we live and have an effect on our daily lives and wellness (Albrarran, 2009; Graham & Choi, 2015; Rosenfield & O'Connor-Petruso, 2014). The next time you walk through campus, stop and watch your classmates walk by. What are they doing? Are they walking by, being aware of their surroundings? Are they having conversations with the people next to them, or do they have their faces buried in the screens of smartphones? While constant overuse of technology can have some detrimental effects (Samaha & Hawi, 2015), using it for health and other matters has proven to be quite beneficial.

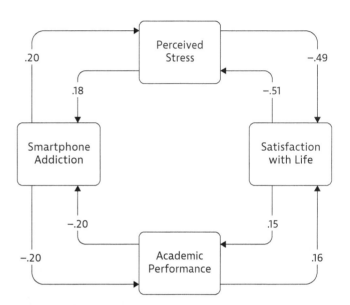

Figure 5.1 *Results of this study showed that smartphone addiction causes stress, and smartphone addiction can also impede academic performance.*

Mobile Devices and Social Media in Health Promotion

Have you thought about the potential uses of social media platforms concerning health promotion and wellness? **Social media** has the potential to reach a large target population with just a few keystrokes. Social media is something that many of us use daily. So why not use it for programming in health promotion and wellness? While specific platforms have faded into obsolescence (Myspace, Vine), others continue to keep going strong (Facebook). Users of social media platforms are constantly updating their statuses on Facebook, uploading pictures to Instagram, tweeting thoughts on Twitter, and taking short videos and photos and adding them to stories on Snapchat. These platforms are readily available on our smartphones and tablets, and many of us will spend quite a bit of time on them (Graham & Choi, 2015).

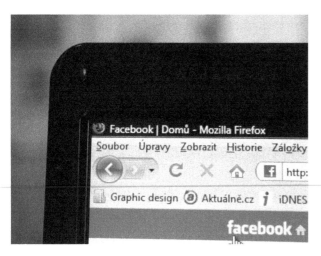

Figure 5.2 *Facebook is an online social media and social networking tool.*

With platforms such as Facebook, individuals are creating groups and programs that promote everything from smoking cessation and weight loss to diabetes foot care programs (Abedin et al., 2017; Napolitano et al., 2017; Naslund et al., 2017). However, the effectiveness of using social media platforms also depends on whether or not someone is motivated intrinsically (internal source) or extrinsically (external source). Individuals who require extrinsic motivation would thrive in a group format on social media (Facebook), while those who are intrinsically motivated would be more successful in an individualized application (MyFitnessPal).

As a social media user, think about how connected you are to your friends, family, and acquaintances and how you're held accountable for what you post on these platforms. There are endless possibilities to utilize Facebook Live within a closed Facebook group. You could provide individuals with information in real time as well as field questions that they may have. Now, take this general idea and apply it to something related to your health. Perhaps it's a weight loss group, or a healthy eating/recipe sharing group. Anything you post in the group is there for everyone to see. Therefore, we become more motivated to follow through with things that we display because we have a support network encouraging us and holding us accountable.

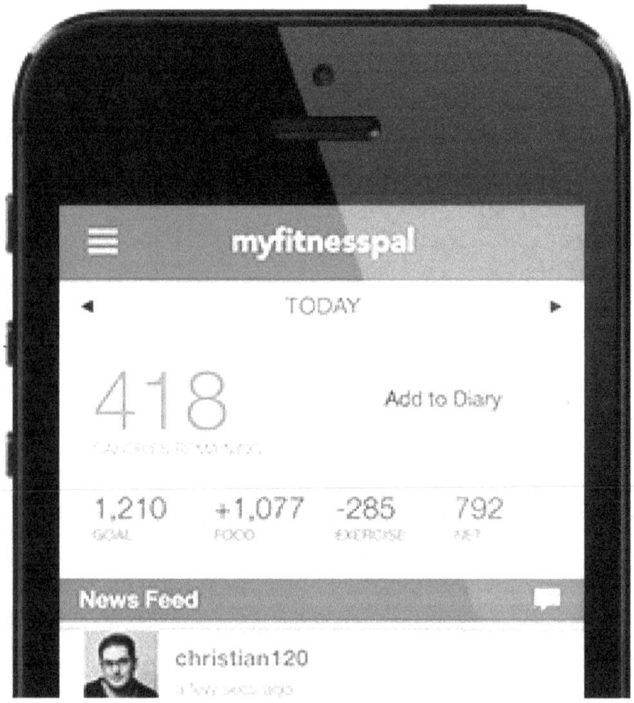

Smartphones and Apps That Motivate Change

Physical

It wasn't until the mid-1990s that mobile phones were being used for technology-based health promotion, and researchers saw some promising results (Bull, 2011). Keep in mind these cutting-edge results involved text message notifications sent to patients regarding appointments and test results. And as with all things technology, it progressed into something much more.

Figure 5.3 *Smartphone application that allows individuals to reach their fitness and health goals all at their fingertips.*

Fast-forward to 2018. We can still receive text message notifications. Still, we also have access to a smartphone app store where we can purchase applications for pretty much anything, including behavior change. Smartphones and applications are a relatively new trend in technology-based health promotion. As we learned in the previous section, individuals can be motivated intrinsically and extrinsically. Those who thrive on intrinsic motivation may prefer to use a smartphone application to track progress and to help them find information to achieve goals.

Things that were difficult 20 years ago, such as getting a child to take their diabetic medication or promoting healthy eating/food selection in young kids, are now made much more attractive. Now, kids with type 1 and type 2 diabetes mellitus can use applications such as "Jerry the Bear and I Got This: An Interactive Story" to help them learn more about their conditions and how to cope with them. The use of gaming applications related to diabetes can remove the stigma often attached to these conditions. This, in turn, can help life for these individuals to become more normalized.

Other behavior changes that could benefit from some type of gaming application include childhood nutrition/eating habits. Using apps such as Awesome Eats and Healthy eating with Diana can help young children identify common fruits and vegetables, help them understand how these foods benefit them, and give them healthy eating tips. Similar to these applications for kids, a variety of behavior change applications are available for adolescents and adults to use. With apps such as MyFitnessPal and My Plate Calorie Counter, users can keep track of eating habits, calorie intake, and calories burned during exercise. Other features available with these applications include workout videos, meal plans, and additional information on healthy eating.

As technology continues to improve, there may even be applications that will cut out the need for quick trips to the doctor and specialist visits altogether. We are currently on the verge of this right now. Many individuals use the WebMD Symptom Checker to "self-diagnose" to forgo or warrant a visit to see a medical professional. A person can enter all their symptoms, and a computer algorithm will inform the individual (in the form of a percentage) what condition(s) they may be suffering from. However, it is essential to proceed with caution when using applications such as these. Many times, patients will self-diagnose themselves with conditions (cancer, Ebola) that can only be found with diagnostic testing. There can also be false-positive conditions reported to an individual because they did not enter all their symptoms or because the computer could not read into what they were telling it. It is still best to consult a doctor before entering all your personal information into an app to have it make your health decisions for you.

Emotional, Spiritual, and Intellectual

Some of the other areas that are addressed by smartphone-based applications include mindfulness and mental health. Apps such as Stop, Breathe & Think, Headspace, Pray as You Go, Lumosity, and Happily fall under the realm of spiritual and intellectual wellness. These applications were developed to help users become more aware of their surroundings, become more mindful, decrease anxiety and stress, be guided through prayer/meditation, and improve critical thinking. These applications offer evidence-based solutions and have users check back in periodically to track their progress. In dealing with emotional wellness, mental health issues, chronic illness, and more, Talkspace Online Therapy provides users with a licensed online therapist with whom to chat. Talkspace Online Therapy is a pay-for-service application that is cheaper than traditional mental health counseling. Prices start at $49/week for direct messaging and $79/week for live chat/video options. This particular application allows individuals to seek advice within the comfort of their own homes. This is an excellent option for those individuals who want to seek counseling but want to avoid some of the negative stigmas that are attached to mental health/mental health counseling.

Financial

Having the ability to track expenses, set up budgets, and have a sense of peace regarding financial situations is yet another dimension of wellness that can be addressed with smartphone applications. Sometimes banks will include a budgeting section in their mobile apps, but they usually are not very user-friendly. For this reason, many applications will help you budget for pretty much everything. If you need to track the inner workings of your retirement plan as well as daily spending, then Personal Capital might be the right app for you.

On the other hand, applications such as Mint and You Need A Budget (YNAB) are great for in-depth/detailed budgeting. If you're just getting started with budgeting, *PocketGuard* is excellent for basic budgeting and linking all your bank accounts. Financial stress is prevalent and, unfortunately, can be crippling for some. Thankfully, the continued improvements and upgrades in smartphone technology and application development can give some individuals both control and peace of mind over their finances.

Occupational and Social

While there are apps dedicated to professional wellness, it's often easier for individuals to use applications such as MyFitnessPal and Fitbit to socialize and improve workplace dynamics. Users of MyFitnessPal and Fitbit can challenge each other to step challenges and nutrition challenges, or they can walk together on their lunch breaks with step goals in mind. Individuals can also set up daily lunchtime meetings with a large group and send an invite out via Google Calendar. Regular lunch meetings give coworkers time to interact with each other and ensure people feel included. This is where occupational wellness begins to transition into social wellness. Work-life balance and meaningful social interaction have become necessities in our day-to-day lives. As with the other six dimensions of wellness, if we lack in either of these areas, it may harm our daily lives.

If you've accepted a new job and it's 12 hours from your home (friends, family, activities) or previous location, you are now in a brand-new place where you don't know anyone. At this point, your coworkers become the first people you meet and often become your first friends in this new place. It's great that you have friends, but the only thing you all have in common may be the workplace. Therefore, all discussions revolve around work. This can become very draining and harm work-life balance. To meet new people, a person can use applications such as Bumble BFF, Friender, The League, Hey!VINA, REALU, and Meet My Dog. All of these apps enable you to meet new people and foster meaningful social relationships. While these applications are helping people meet each other, it should be noted that a person should always make their safety a top priority. Therefore, it is commonly recommended that before meeting someone, you still do a search using TruthFinder (online background check) as well as browse their social media accounts to make sure they are a real person.

Social wellness is also a common issue with new mothers. Postpartum depression and lack of human interaction (besides with the baby) can harm the new mother's social wellness. Applications such as Peanut help new moms find/meet other new moms. The app takes the child's age and location to support the new mom finding postpartum friends to socialize with. The application also utilizes a platform to discuss serious/severe diagnoses such as postpartum depression (PPD) and more light-hearted concerns about diaper types and diaper services. In regards to PPD, there is an application, PPD ACT (Apple iOS only), that is more like a research study. The application has users answer a set of questions regarding PPD. While there is not a diagnosis provided, using this app can help scientists and practitioners treat PPD more effectively.

Wearable Technology and Other Information

If you look at the wrist/hand of the person sitting next to you, you may notice a sporty-looking watch or a strange-looking ring. These watches and bracelets are part of an increasingly popular wearable technology market. These trackers are convenient because they can record movement, track sleep, measure heart rate, and estimate caloric expenditure without extra equipment, such as the chest straps found on so many heart rate monitors of yesterday. They are also functional and efficient because they serve the dual purpose of tracking your movement and vital signs, all while looking like a fashion accessory.

While they are quite trendy, research has found they do not work as well as we once thought (Gonzalez, 2017). Many of the devices do not track time, calorie expenditure, steps taken, and heart rate accurately. An individual may consume too many calories because their fitness tracker states they have burned 7,000 calories in a day when in all actuality, they have only burned 4,000 calories. This does not mean you should stop wearing your device if you own one. According to Gonzalez (2017), some of the current research is relatively old in terms of technology studied. As mentioned earlier, this happens quite often with anything technology related. As newer models appear on the market, their accompanying software is being improved to account for these discrepancies.

The overwhelmingly positive aspect of these fitness trackers is that many of them have built-in support systems to encourage users to stay active and healthy. For example, Fitbit has a section on their website called "Fitbit Stories—Find Your Reason." This provides individuals with success stories from real Fitbit users and how they were motivated to make changes in their lives. Another motivator Fitbit offers within their application is the step challenge. Individuals challenge each other to take x number of steps in a day or week. This keeps individuals up and active so that they can potentially beat their competitors' step count. While accurate wearable technology is still in its infancy, it still provides users with a tool to lead healthier lives.

Telemedicine

With access, equity, quality, and cost-effectiveness being the major issues affecting health care in both developed and less developed countries, it is more important than ever that health educators are able to communicate and exchange information in a variety of ways. Modern Information and communication technologies (ICTs) are revolutionizing how we seek and exchange information. Technologies such as computers, internet, smart-phones, wearable technology all have a great potential to help address contemporary global health problems (WHO, 2010).

Telemedicine is a term that was coined in the early 1970's, which means "healing at a distance" (Strehle & Shabde, 2006). The WHO (1998) states that telemedicine is "the delivery of health care services, where distance is a critical factor, by all health care professionals using information and communication technologies for the exchange of valid information for diagnosis, treatment and prevention of disease and injuries, research and evaluation, and for the continuing education of health care providers, all in the interests of advancing the health of individuals and their communities". The main purposes of telemedicine is to provide clinical support by overcoming geographical barriers, and connecting users who are not in the same physical location (WHO, 1998). Over the past decade there has been a rapid increase in new developments for health-care delivery, with written records being transferred to digital methods, and a drop in cost for information technology it has sparked health care providers and organizations to implement new and more efficient ways of providing care (Craig & Patterson, 2005; Currell et al., 2000). The internet has further accelerated the pace of these advancements and expanded telemedicine to encompass web-based applications like teleconsultations and web-conferences through the internet (Craig & Patterson, 2005).

Telehealth

Telehealth is a term that has been used interchangeably with telemedicine, however, they have some differences. Telehealth encompasses a broad variety of technologies to assist individuals in health, health education services, and public health information. Telemedicine often is only focused on remote clinical care, while telehealth is a broader scope of health care services (wellness coaching, nutrition services, health coach, etc.) (American Academy of Family Physicians (AAFP), 2020).

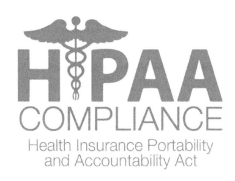

Figure 5.4 *HIPPA: Health Insurance Portability and Accountability Act.*

Technology Trends in Healthcare and HIPPA

In the past 20 years, healthcare has grown by leaps and bounds concerning the use of computer-based technology. Healthcare providers can utilize electronic medical records to increase their efficiency and effectiveness (Acharya, Shimpi, Mahnke, Mathias, & Ye, 2017). Along with using electronic medical records, many healthcare providers are utilizing patient portals to provide a more patient-centered care model, which means they focus more on the individual patient when making choices regarding care (Safadi, Chan, Dawes, Roper, & Faraj, 2014).

These electronic medical records are incredibly beneficial to the patients, as it provides them with their medical history and billing information as well as future scheduled appointments. Each portal is password protected for each patient to maintain security, the protection of patient information. With a decreased paper trail, mistakes and Health Insurance Portability Accountability Act (HIPAA) violations may become a distant memory.

It is no question that technology is undoubtedly changing the way we function as a society. Digital natives, or individuals who were born into the digital world, are going to foster the field of health promotion and wellness in a new era. In doing so, we will hopefully see the end of the digital divide.

Review Questions

1. Define health technology. Why is health technology important in health promotion?

2. Which smartphone app discussed in this chapter could potential violate an individual's HIPPAA rights? What about apps that are not discussed in this chapter? Explain.

3. Explain the similarities in how technology can be used for the physical dimension of wellness and the mental/emotional dimension of wellness?

4. Explain the pros and cons of health technology as discussed in this chapter.

Case Scenario

You have been hired by the local YMCA to implement a smoking cessation program within the community. You are given a $10,000 yearly budget to help with the costs of the program. After doing some research, you have discovered using technology may be a way to help with smoking cessation. What will you purchase with your money to help the participants in the program? How will these purchases help someone stop smoking? When determining where to spend your money, think about things like limited access to the Internet, lack of mobile devices, motivation, socioeconomic status, etc.

Critical Thinking Questions

1. You have been asked to teach a health and technology course for college students in your department. What aspects of health and technology will you focus on for the students? What activity will you create and have the students participate in to understand the pros and cons of health technology?

2. You are working for a company whose employees are mostly sedentary. As the worksite wellness coordinator, you have been hired to make employees more active. The problem is they are only allowed two 15-minute breaks and a 1-hour lunch. How could you get the employees to be more active using technology?

3. For college students, social media can be a major distraction, especially when they are in class. How can professors and instructors incorporate the use of social media into their classrooms? For example, how could your health and wellness professor use technology or social media to spice up the classroom lesson? Explain using some of the applications from this chapter.

Activities

1. If a friend, family member, or classmate has one of these pieces of technology on, ask them the following questions:

   a. What do you like about your fitness tracker/smartwatch?
   b. Has this piece of technology helped you achieve your goals?
   c. How much was the item? Was it worth the money? Why or why not?

2. Download one of the applications discussed in the chapter (or find one of your own) and explore it.

   a. What are the things that make this an excellent application to use?
   b. What are some shortcomings of the application?
   c. Do you think smartphone applications are useful for behavior?

3. Using Snapchat, purchase a filter (or don't) and create a snap story that involves you promoting awareness related to one of the following areas: testicular cancer awareness, smoking/dipping cessation, or healthy eating habits.

   a. Would this type of promotion activity be useful? Why or why not?
   b. What are some strengths of this platform?
   c. What are some weaknesses of this platform?

Weblinks

https://www.who.int/health-technology-assessment/about/healthtechnology/en/

The World Health Organization (WHO)

Use this site to understand the use of health technology and assessment. This site gives information on country capacities regarding health technology as well as tools and resources to help support decision makers with health and technology.

https://www.nlm.nih.gov/nichsr/hta101/ta10103.html

National Library of Medicine

The National Information Center on Health Services Research and Health Care Technology (NICHSR) looks at the origins of technology, early health technology, and several factors that reinforce the market for health technology.

https://www.cdwg.com/content/cdwg/en/industries/healthcare-technology.html

CDWG People Who Get It

This website looks at today's technology-focused landscape and a variety of different dependable health technologies.

https://www.springer.com/journal/12553

Springer Health and Technology Journal

The *Health and Technology* research journal is the first truly cross-disciplinary journal on issues related to health technologies, addressing all professions relating to health care and health technology.

References

Abedin, T., Mamun, M. A., Lasker, M. A. A., Ahmed, S. W., Shommu, N., Rumana, N., & Turin, T. C. (2017). Social media as a platform for information about diabetes foot care: A study of Facebook groups. *Canadian Journal of Diabetes, 41,* 97–101.

Acharya, A., Shimpi, N., Mahnke, A., Mathias, R., & Ye, Z. (2017). Medical care providers' perspectives on dental information needs in electronic health records. *The Journal of the American Dental Association, 148(5),* 328–337.

Albrarran, A. B. (2009). Young Latinos use of mobile phones: A cross-cultural study. *Revista de Communication, 8,* 95–108.

American Academy of Family Physicians (AAFP). (2020). What's the difference between telemedicine and telehealth? Retrieved from http://www.who.int/goe/publications/goe_telemedicine_2010.pdf

American Diabetes Association. (2018). *Facebook.* Retrieved from facebook.com/americandiabetesassociation

Bull, S. (2011). *Technology-based health promotion.* Thousand Oaks, CA: Sage Publications.

Craig, J., Patterson, V. (2000). Introduction to the practice of telemedicine. *Journal of Telemedicine and Telecare, 11*(1):3–9.

Currell, R., et al. (2000). Telemedicine versus face to face patient care: effects on professional practice and health care outcomes. *Cochrane Database of Systematic Reviews*, Issue 2. Art. No.: CD002098.

Fitbit Stories (2017). *Find your reason.* Retrieved from https://stories.fitbit.com/

Graham, R., & Choi, K. S. (2015). Explaining African-American cell phone usage through the social shaping of technology approach. *Journal of African American Studies, 20,* 19–34.

Gonzalez, R. (2017). *Science says fitness trackers don't work. Wear one anyway. Wired.* Retrieved from https://www.wired.com/story/science-says-fitness-trackers-dont-work-wear-one-anyway/

Group Internet Platform Inc. *Talkspace Online Therapy* (Version 7.1). [Mobile application software]. Retrieved from http://itunes.apple.com/

Happily, Inc. (2018). Happily (Version 2.5.3). [Mobile application software]. Retrieved from http://itunes.apple.com

Kreuter, M. W., & Strecher, V. J. (1996). Do tailored behavior change messages enhance the effectiveness of health risk appraisal? Results from a randomized trial. *Health Education Research, 11*(1), 97–105.

LIVESTRONG.COM. (2018). MyPlate Calorie Counter (Version 5.13.1). [Mobile application software]. Retrieved from http://itunes.apple.com

Mútua General de Catalunya. (2018). Healthy eating with Diana (Version 2.2). [Mobile application software]. Retrieved from http://itunes.apple.com

MyFitnessPal.com (2018). MyFitnessPal (Version 7.31). [Mobile application software]. Retrieved from http://itunes.apple.com

Napolitano, M. A., Whiteley, J. A., Mavredes, M. N., Faro, J., DiPietro, L., Hayman, L. L., Neighbors, C. J., & Simmens, S. (2017). Using social media to deliver weight loss programming to young adults: Design and rationale for the Healthy Body Healthy U (HBHU) trial. *Contemporary Clinical Trials. 60,* 1–13.

Naslund, J. A., Kim, S. J., Aschbrenner, K. A., McCulloch, L. J., Brunette, M. F., Dallery, J., Bartels, S. J., & Marsch, L. A. (2017). Systemic review of social media interventions for smoking cessation. *Addictive Behaviors, 73,* 81–93.

Rosenfield, B., & O'Connor-Petruso, S. A. (2014). East vs. West: A comparison of mobile phone use by Chinese and American college students. *College Student Journal, 48*(2), 312–321.

Safadi, H., Chan, D., Dawes, M., Roper, M., & Faraj, S. (2014). Open-source health information technology: A case study of electronic medical records. *Health Policy and Technology, 4,* 14–28.

Samaha, M., & Hawi, N. (2015). Relationships among smartphone addiction, stress, academic performance, and satisfaction with life. *Computers in Human Behavior, 57,* 321–325.

Sproutel Inc. (2017). Jerry the Bear (Version 1.20). [Mobile application software]. Retrieved from http://itunes.apple.com

Stop, Breathe & Think. (2018). Stop, Breath & Think (Version 4.4). [Mobile application software]. Retrieved from http://itunes.apple.com

Strehle, E.M., Shabde, N. (2006). One hundred years of telemedicine: Does this new technology have a place in paediatrics? *Archives of Disease in Childhood, 91*(12):956–959.

WebMD. (2017). WebMD symptom checker. Retrieved from https://symptoms.webmd.com/default.htm#/info

Whole Kids Foundation. (2016). Awesome Eats (Version 1.4) [Mobile application software]. Retrieved from http://itunes.apple.com

University of California, Berkley's Lawrence Hall of Science. (2017). I Got This: An Interactive Story (Version 2.0). [Mobile application software]. Retrieved from http://itunes.apple.com

Van Cura, L. J., Jensen, N. M., Greist, J. H., Lewis, W. R., & Frey, S. R. (1975). Venereal disease. Interviewing and teaching by computer. *American Journal of Public Health, 65*(11), 1159–1164.

WHO. (1998). *A health telematics policy in support of WHO's Health-For-All strategy for global health development: report of the WHO group consultation on health telematics,* 11–16 December, Geneva, 1997. Geneva, World Health Organization, 1998.

WHO (2010). Telemedicine: Opportunities and developments in member states. Global Observatory for eHealth Series, 2. Retrieved from http://www.who.int/goe/publications/goe_telemedicine_2010.pdf

Credits

CHAPTER 6

A Background to Theory and Planning Models in Health Education and Promotion

CHAPTER KEY

Authentic Learning: **using problem-solving of real-life scenarios to explore and discuss content and concepts.**

Knowledge: **the theoretical or practical understanding of a concept.**

Reflection: **contemplation or meditation.**

Practice: **applications of ideas or concepts.**

Collaboration: **working with content from other organizations or peers.**

Leadership: **the act of leading a group or organization.**

Chapter Objectives

After reading this chapter and answering the questions at the end of the chapter, you will be able to:

- **Differentiate** between health-promoting and health-hindering behaviors (*knowledge, reflection*).

- **Apply** concepts and theories of health education and health promotion (*authentic learning, knowledge, reflection, practice, collaboration & leadership*).

- **Explain** the importance of theory in health education and health promotion (*knowledge, reflection*).

- **Identify** behavior change theories and their components (*knowledge, reflection, practice, collaboration & leadership*).

Chapter Links to the Areas of Responsibility of a Health Educator/Health Promotion Professional

- Area of Responsibility I: Assessment of Needs Capacity

- Area of Responsibility II: Planning

- Area of Responsibility III: Implementation

- Area of Responsibility V: Advocacy

- Area of Responsibility VI: Communication

- Area of Responsibility VII: Leadership and Management

- Area of Responsibility VIII: Ethics and Professionalism

Introduction

As noted in previous chapters, health promotion and wellness has evolved dramatically since the earliest humans and is continuously changing the way we advocate for health across the globe. As the profession has grown, so has the number of intrapersonal, interpersonal, and community theories as well as program models used by health education specialists. This chapter introduces primary elements such as *theory, model, concept, construct,* and *variable.* Each theory and model presented in this chapter will use these primary elements to either design interventions or aid in behavior change. This chapter will expose you to just a few theories and models used in health education and health promotion. However, throughout your career, you will be exposed to a wide variety of theories and models that stem from those presented here. Please note that not all theories and models are covered in this chapter.

Primary Elements

When discussing behavior change, both theories and models are essential to understand. The term "**theory**" has been addressed by several individuals over the years to compile a thorough definition. In 2005, Rimer and Glanz defined theory as "a set of concepts, definitions, and propositions that explain or predict these events or situations by illustrating the relationships between variables" (p. 11). Overall, theories are a way of explaining complex phenomena.

With behavior change theories, we discuss the term "theory" to identify what may, or may not, affect an individual to make a lifestyle change. The term "**concepts**," presented in the definition of theory, are the ideas or "building blocks" behind the theory (Rimer & Glanz, 2005). **Constructs** are concepts that have been developed and defined for use in theory. We use "variables" to measure the degree to which the likelihood of the behavior change will occur. **Variables** are the "quantitative measurement of a construct" (Rimer & Glanz, 2005). As you will see in this chapter, each behavior change theory and model has its unique constructs and variables.

The term "theory" is often confused with the term "**model**." According to Rimer and Glanz (2005), "models draw on several theories to help people understand a specific problem in a particular setting or context" (p. 11). Models are more generalized and not always as detailed as theories because they only represent the process, not explain it (Chaplin & Krawiec, 1979).

The Importance of Theory and Planning Models

Theories and models are essential components in health promotion because they are the basis for assessing the four major components of behavior change practices: needs assessment, program planning, program implementation, and program evaluation. More specifically, theories and models address the following: (1) reasons why people are not behaving in healthy ways; (2) identify information needed before developing an intervention; (3) provide a conceptual framework for selecting constructs to build the intervention; (4) give insight into how best to deliver the intervention; and (5) identify measurements needed to evaluate the intervention's impact (Crosby, Kegler, & DiClemente, 2009; Glanz, Rimer, & Viswanath, 2008; Salazar, Crosby, & DiClemente, 2013).

Throughout the rest of this chapter, you will see that the behavior change theories will be introduced based on their grouping of socio-ecological, intrapersonal, interpersonal, and community. Additionally, two health promotion and wellness planning models will be discussed.

Behavior Change Theories

As noted earlier, there are many different types of theories used for a variety of different situations and events. Behavior change theories "specify the relationships among causal processes operating both within and across levels of analysis" (McLeroy, Steckler, Goodman, & Burdine, 1992, p. 3). Behavior change theories can guide health educators in understanding why people behave in specific ways. This chapter will discuss **behavior change theories** such as the health belief model, transtheoretical model, theory of planned behavior, social cognitive theory, diffusion of innovation theory, community readiness model, and socio-ecological approach. This chapter will also identify the previously mentioned theories as intrapersonal, interpersonal, or community.

Intrapersonal Theories

Intrapersonal theories are theories whose constructs are based on what the individual values. Intrapersonal factors include knowledge, attitudes, beliefs, motivation, self-concept, developmental history, experience, and skills. Individual-level theories are presented below (Rimer & Glanz, 2005). In this chapter, the intrapersonal theories will be discussed (health belief model, transtheoretical model of change, and theory of planned behavior).

The Health Belief Model

The **health belief model (HBM)** was proposed by a team of social psychologists in the 1950s to explain participation in preventive health behaviors (Hochbaum, 1958; Kegeles, Kirscht, Haefner, & Rosenstock, 1965; Rosenstock, 1966, 1974). The United States was experiencing a health crisis associated with too few physicians and high healthcare costs, which resulted in the insufficient treatment of patients (Derryberry, 2004). The idea of disease prevention was introduced to

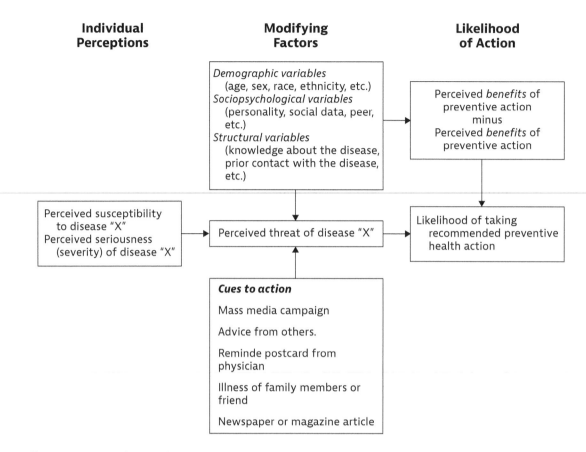

Figure 6.1 *The Health Belief Model Constructs.*

reduce the number of patients who needed to see a physician so cost and treatment levels could return to their original levels. The HBM is used as a tool to predict why, or why not, an individual takes part in preventive behaviors associated with disease prevention (Rosenstock, 1966).

The HBM is a continuum theory, and the constructs are all dependent on the individual's beliefs that the behavior change will result in something of value to them (Rosenstock, 1966). For example, a desire to avoid illness to regain health status and live longer is usually of importance to most individuals.

The six original constructs all relate to personal beliefs for behavior change: perceived benefits, perceived barriers, perceived susceptibility, perceived seriousness, perceived threat, and cues to action (Rosenstock, 1974). **Perceived benefits** are the individual's beliefs about whether this impact is intrinsically positive or negative (Janz & Becker, 1984). If it is inherently positive, or highly beneficial to them, then the behavior is more likely to occur than if the individual views the impact as less favorable. **Perceived barriers** are the obstacles that must be overcome to make a successful behavior change. Perceived barriers must be considered because they could be obstacles when making changes in behavior that could outweigh the positive benefits (Rosenstock, 1974). When this happens, and the barriers outweigh the benefits, it is less likely that the individual will be able to make the behavior change.

Together, **perceived susceptibility** to disease and **perceived seriousness** of a condition contribute to the **perceived threat** of disease (Becker, Drachman, & Kirscht, 1974). Perceived susceptibility is the belief about how likely it is that someone will get the disease, while perceived seriousness is how severely they believe the disease will affect them. According to the HBM, the greater the perceived susceptibility and severity are, the higher the perceived threat will be. This will increase the likelihood that the recommended behavior change will occur (Janz & Becker, 1984). Perceived threat acts as a central construct to bridge beliefs and actions.

Cues to action are the daily encounters one may experience that could remind them that they are at risk for disease (Janz & Becker, 1984). For example, if you see a television advertisement about smoking, it could trigger thoughts about lung and mouth cancer, chronic obstructive pulmonary disease (COPD), stroke, etc., if the individual is a smoker.

In addition to the constructs of the health belief model, some variables may impact behavior change (demographic, socio-psychological, and structural). These variables impact behavior change when an individual has a specific risk factor for a condition/disease. Ultimately, this would increase the individual's **perceived threat,** which would increase their likelihood of acting to prevent disease (Keida, 2016).

The Transtheoretical Model (Stages of Change)

The **transtheoretical model of change (TMC)** is a stage theory that describes individuals' motivation and readiness to change a behavior (Rimer & Glanz, 2005). Prochaska developed the TMC in 1979 following his work in psychotherapy. The TMC has seven stages (pre-contemplation, contemplation, preparation, action, maintenance, termination, and relapse). Based on the individual's intentions and behaviors, it is clear as to which stage they are in within this model. Unlike the fluid nature of continuum theories, such as the HBM, the steps in the TMC make it more transparent as to where the individual is in the behavior change process.

The furthest stage an individual can be in from making a behavior change is **pre-contemplation.** The pre-contemplation stage is when the individual has not considered making a behavior change and will not for at least 6 months (Rimer & Glanz, 2005). Generally, the individual may not even believe there is a problem with their current behavior. In Prochaska and DiClemente's (1982) research on the psychotherapy of smoking cessation, pre-contemplation is demonstrated by the smokers continuing the behavior because they have no intention to quit. According to Prochaska and Velicer (1997), this could be due to discouragement from a previous

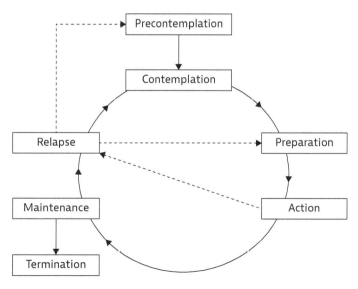

Figure 6.2 *The Transtheoretical Model: The Journey Through Stages.*

unsuccessful attempt or lack of knowledge regarding the risks of their behavior to disease (Prochaska & DiClemente, 1982).

The second stage of **contemplation** is when the individual does recognize there is a problem with their current behavior and is considering making a behavior change. They have not yet committed to making a change but are aware of the pros and cons of making the behavior change (Prochaska & Velicer, 1997). It is expected that within the next 6 months, the change will occur (Rimer & Glanz, 2005). **Preparation,** the third stage, is when the individual is actively preparing to make a behavior change. They have not yet practiced the new behavior, but a plan is being developed to make the change within the next 30 days (Rimer & Glanz, 2005). Actions that may have been taken within the year prior to this stage include enrolling in a health education class, having conversations with a doctor, consulting a counselor, purchasing products needed to assist with the change, etc. (Prochaska & Velicer, 1997).

When the actual change is being practiced, it is called **action**. The individual has been taking measures to reduce disease risk for less than 6 months (Rimer & Glanz, 2005). According to scientists, not all actions would be considered significant for this stage. With smoking cessation, there would be an actual cigarette count performed to see if the action was sufficient (Prochaska & Velicer, 1997). Once the behavior has been practiced for more than 6 months, the individual would move into the **maintenance stage** (Rimer & Glanz, 2005). There are still triggers for the old behavior, and the individual is still actively working towards implementing the new behavior. The final stage is **termination**. In this stage, there is no temptation to return to the old behavior, and the individuals have 100 percent self-efficacy in the new behavior (Prochaska & Velicer, 1997).

As indicated in the image, **relapse** can occur, disrupting the order of the stages and stepping backward in the behavior change process.

Theory of Planned Behavior

The **theory of planned behavior (TPB)** is an extension of the theory of reasoned action (Ajzen & Fishbein, 1980; Fishbein & Ajzen, 1975). The TPB predicts and explains a wide range of health behaviors and intentions, including substance use, condom use, leisure, and exercise, among many others. The TPB states that behavioral achievement depends on both **motivation** (**intention**) and **ability** (**behavioral control**; LaMorte, 2019). It distinguishes among three types of beliefs: behavioral, normative, and control. The TPB is comprised of six constructs that represent an individual's actual control over the behavior (LaMorte, 2019): (1) **attitudes** refer to one's favorable or unfavorable assessments of the behavior at hand; (2) **behavioral intentions** are the motivational factors that influence the behavior; the stronger the intention, the more likely the behavior will be performed; (3) **subjective norms** are beliefs about whether others, such as peers, approve or disapprove of the behavior; (4) **social norms** are standard behaviors and considered normative in a group of people; (5) **perceived power** is when factors hinder the performance of a behavior and contributes to an individual's perceived behavioral control over those factors; and (6) **perceived behavioral control** refers to one's perceptions of the ease or difficulty of performing a behavior (LaMorte, 2019). (see **Figure 6.3**).

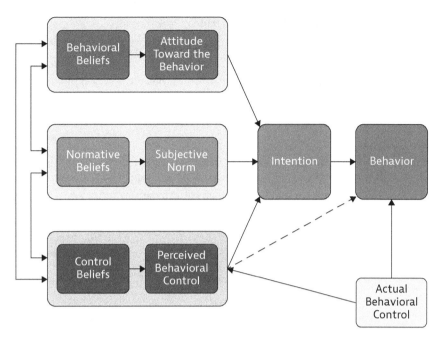

Figure 6.3 *The Theory of Planned Behavior's Six Constructs.*

Interpersonal Theories

Interpersonal-level theories assume that individuals are influenced by their social environments. "The opinions, thoughts, behavior, advice, and support of the people surrounding an individual influence his or her feelings and behavior, and the individual has a reciprocal effect on those people" (Rimer & Glanz, 2005, p. 19). Social relationships, such as those with friends, peers, family members, coworkers, etc., can have the most significant influence on an individual's health behaviors and actions. A critical theory that describes learning as a shared interaction among an individual's environment, cognitive processes, and behavior is known as the social cognitive theory (Parcel et al., 1987).

Social Cognitive Theory

Once known as **social learning theory, social cognitive theory (SCT)** was relabeled by Bandura in 1986 (Bandura, 1986). SCT focuses on rewards, punishments, and reinforcements and how these contribute to learning. SCT explains how individuals acquire and maintain behavior while taking into consideration other factors such as their environment and past experiences. These past experiences can influence the use of reinforcements, expectations, and expectancies, which all impact how one will engage or engages in a particular behavior. The goal of SCT is to explain how people regulate their behavior through control and reinforcement to achieve goal-directed behavior that can be maintained over time (LaMorte, 2019). **Table 6.1** provides a summary of the constructs and how to apply the constructs in a health promotion intervention.

Table 6.1 SOCIAL COGNITIVE THEORY CONSTRUCTS AND EXAMPLES

Construct	Definition	Application
Behavioral Capability	Knowledge and skills needed to influence behavior.	Provide information specific to behavior change.
Outcome Expectations	Individuals' beliefs about the results of the action.	Model positive outcomes.
Outcome Expectancies	The value one places on a given outcome, incentives, represents the fundamental idea that most individuals will not choose to do a task when they expect to fail.	Present outcomes of change that have applied, functional meaning.
Environments and Situations	Provide an ecological framework for behavior change. Perceptions of the environment.	Provide opportunities to practice healthy behavior. Provide support, correct misperceptions.
Observational Learning	Individual's beliefs based on observing others.	Identify role models to emulate.
Reinforcement	Responses to a person's behavior that increase or decrease the chance of reoccurrence.	Provide incentives, rewards, praise, encourage self-rewards.
Self-Efficacy	Belief in one's ability to perform a task.	Point out strengths, use persuasion and encouragement.
Self-Control	Personal regulation of goal-directed behavior.	Decision; self-monitoring; goal setting; problem-solving.
Managing Emotional Arousal	Strategies or tactics to deal with emotional stimuli	Training in problem-solving and stress management.

Community Theories

Community theories refer to behavior change approaches or participation in health behavior that can be impacted by the individual aspects of an organization, such as norms and official policies. Community behavior change models are different than personal behavior change models because rather than focusing on a single lifestyle change, the health promotion specialist must consider starting a program, changing policy, or alerting personnel roles (Rimer & Glanz, 2005). Two community theories that will be discussed are diffusion theory and the community readiness model.

Diffusion of Innovation Theory

The **diffusion theory (DT)**, or **diffusion of innovations theory**, is a stage theory that "addresses how new ideas, products, and social practices spread within an organization, community, or society" (Rimer & Glanz, 2005, p. 34). In the health field, it is imperative to understand how ideas are spread to determine how new medical information, practices, invention, etc., will be disseminated. This information can improve the quality of life more quickly and even be lifesaving.

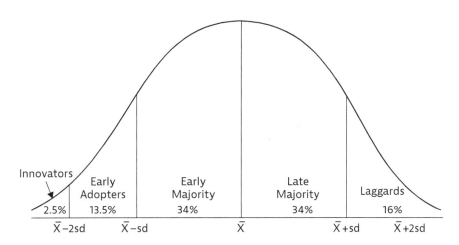

Figure 6.4 *The Diffusion of Innovation: Categories of Adopters.*

The process by which individuals adopt a new idea, product, or social practice can be described using a bell-shaped curve (**Figure 6.4**). Those who are exposed to the original idea, product, or social practice are called adopters and fall into one of the five stages. The rate at which they first engage with the new practice is what categorizes them.

Innovators adopt innovation first. Generally, they can be considered "venturesome, independent, risky, and daring" (Cottrell, Girvan, McKenzie, & Seabert, 2015, p. 117). **Early adopters** are also quick to adopt innovation but are not the first. Due to their independent but also slightly cautious nature, early adopters are looked at as opinion leaders (Cottrell, Girvan, McKenzie, & Seabert, 2015).

The **early** and **late majority** contain most of the decision-making group. The early majority are usually interested in the innovation but need additional motivation to make the change. In contrast, the late majority, consisting of skeptics, are not involved in the innovation but may see practical aspects of the innovation after others (innovators, early adopters, and early majority) have already adopted it and put it to use. The final group to get involved in innovation, if they ever commit, are the **laggards**. They lack interest in innovation and are in no rush to adopt.

Community Readiness Model

The **community readiness model (CRM)** is a tool used to determine at what stage of readiness a group of people are in to implement a program (Edwards, Jumper-Thurman, Plested, Oetting, & Swanson, 2000). Similar to the TMC, the CRM is a stage theory. Determining a community's readiness to change based on the stage they're in is much more evident than in a continuum. However, as previously discussed, community models require the attention and commitment of a group of people, not just an individual. When considering this particular model, determining the stages of readiness to change is dependent on the entire organization. As shown in **Table 6.2**, the CRM consists of nine steps.

Table 6.2 STAGES OF THE COMMUNITY READINESS MODEL (EDWARDS ET AL., 2000)

Stage	Description of Stage
No Awareness	As a whole, the community and leaders do not recognize the issue as a problem.
Denial	Although there is the recognition that the problem exists, the community and leaders may not see it as a problem in their community. There may be feelings of inability to help the problem.
Vague Awareness	Community members and/or leaders may recognize the problem exists locally but fail to do anything about it. There is a lack of motivation among the community and leaders to make a change.
Preplanning	There is recognition among the community and leaders that there is a problem, and some action has been taken. However, the actions that have been put into place, such as a task force, lack detail and planning.
Preparation	The planning process has started, and a detailed plan of action is being developed based on data collected from the community. Leadership is fully involved.
Initiation	The plan has been implemented but is still being evaluated for quality control. Staff is being trained, and a majority of the community is involved.
Stabilization	Programs are running and considered stable. Staff have experience and begin to troubleshoot problems based on formative evaluation strategies. The community has a positive outlook on the program. There is no growth at this time.
Confirmation/ Expansion	Programs have set standards (activities and policies) by which they are expected to run. The community and leaders support the expansion of the program. Changes, based on summative evaluation methods, are being made to improve the effectiveness of the program. Efforts are in place to seek resources for expansion. Ongoing data collection is taking place.
Professionalism	Detailed knowledge related to the prevalence and risk factors of the problem exists. Highly trained staff make new efforts to target high-risk groups as well as the general population. Programs are continually being evaluated.

Copyright © 2000 by Ruth W. Edwards, Maria Leonora G. Comello, Kathleen J. Kelly, Barbara A. Plested, Pamela Jumper Thurman, and Michael D. Slater.

Socio-Ecological Approach

To understand the multitude of factors that impact behavior, we must first look at the **socio-ecological approach** (sometimes referred to as the socio-ecological perspective). The socio-ecological approach provides an underlying concept that behavior has multiple levels of influence. This approach "emphasizes the interaction between, and the interdependence of, factors within and across all levels of a health problem" (Rimer & Glanz, 2005, p. 10). Individuals are influenced in many ways through family, friends, and communities they are a part of, otherwise known as social context. **Social context** is defined as "the sociocultural forces that shape people's day-to-day experiences and that directly and indirectly affect health and behavior" (Burke, Joseph, Pasick, & Barker, 2009, p. 56S). The socio-ecological approach provides the opportunity for intervention aimed at the multiple levels of influence, which include (1) intrapersonal level, (2) interpersonal level, (3) institutional/organizational level, (4) community level, and (5) public policy level (**Figure 6.5**).

The **individual (intrapersonal) level** of the socio-ecological approach looks at the individual's character-istics, such as knowledge, attitudes, beliefs, skills, and motivation. This level also focuses on one's self-concept, age, gender, and genetics. Take smoking, for example. An individual at this level may be aware of the risks associated with smoking, and *some* have tried to quit.

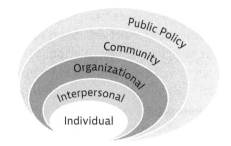

Figure 6.5 *Socio-Ecological Model.*

The **interpersonal level** of the socio-ecological approach looks at an individual's social support, social networks, social norms, and the environment. At this level, many smokers have been encouraged by their social networks, such as family, friends, and even physicians, to quit. Some may try to get support from an organization to stop.

The **institutional/organizational level** looks at the educational system, one's access to healthcare and services, and social interactions. Many universities now have smoke-free cam-puses. Many local parks are smoke-free; these organizations have developed policies to prohibit smoking on the property or grounds.

At the **community level**, we look at one's living and working conditions, public safety, local public health, housing, and economic development. Many towns have local ordinances that prohibit smoking in public places.

The **public policy** level focuses on federal, state, and local policies/laws. Many countries have clean air acts that aim to limit smoking. We often see many government-funded public service announcements aimed at reducing tobacco use or interventions for quitting.

Planning Models for Health Promotion and Wellness

Health promotion programs use conceptual frameworks such as theories and models to provide a well-thought-out and planned intervention for communities, organizations, and individuals. "Planning an effective program is more difficult than implementing it. Planning, implementing, and evaluating programs are all interrelated, but good planning skills are the prerequisite to programs worthy of evaluation" (Minelli & Breckon, 2009, p. 137). There are a variety of different models that can help a health educator in creating an effective program. This section will focus on two specific models, the generalized model and the PRECEDE-PROCEED model.

Generalized Model

The **generalized model (GM)** teaches the basic principles of planning and evaluation for the health professions. The GM is not a new model: it is merely a composite of most planning models. The GM includes five essential elements: (1) assessing needs, (2) setting goals and objectives, (3) developing an intervention, (4) implementing the response, and (5) evaluating the results (**Figure 6.6**). This type of pre-planning allows health educators to answer critical questions and have a good understanding of the community they are targeting. **Assessing needs** requires planners to collect and analyze data on their target population. This means planners will find out as much as they can about the target population because every community is unique and may require different resources or health needs. When **setting goals and objectives**, the planners ask "What will be accomplished? What do we intend to do, and how will we do it?" **Developing interventions** is necessary for determining how the goals and objectives will be achieved. **Implementing the interventions** will put the developed intervention into action to aid in effective behavior change. **Evaluating results** then improves the quality of the program/intervention and determine its effectiveness.

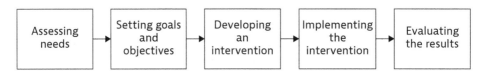

Figure 6.6 *The Generalized Model for Program Planning.*

PRECEDE-PROCEED Model

The best known and most frequently used planning model is the **PRECEDE-PROCEED model**. PRECEDE is an acronym for **p**redisposing, **r**einforcing, and **e**nabling **c**onstructs in **e**ducational/**e**cological **d**iagnosis and **e**valuation. PROCEED stands for **p**olicy, **r**egulatory, and **o**rganizational **c**onstructs in **e**ducational and **e**nvironmental **d**evelopment (Green & Kreuter, 2005). The primary approach to this model is to work first with the final consequences and then work backward to the causes. In other words, begin to identify the outcome, determine what causes it, and then design the intervention (McKenzie, Neiger, & Thackeray, 2013). The PRECEDE-PROCEED model consists of eight phases used for creating interventions (**Figure 6.7**).

Phase 1 is known as **social assessment**, which defines the quality of life within the priority population. Quality of life can consist of achievement, alienation, comfort, crime, discrimination, happiness, self-esteem, unemployment, and welfare (McKenzie, Neiger, & Thackeray, 2013).

Phase 2 is known as the **epidemiological assessment**, where analysis of data can identify the health needs of the priority population. The data includes mortality, morbidity, and disability rates as well as genetic, behavioral, and environmental factors (Green & Kreuter, 2005). In this phase, it is essential to rank the health problems to gain insight into what the program needs to plan.

Phase 3 is the **educational and ecological assessment**, identifying factors and behaviors that could be influencing an individual's behaviors. Three main categories used to identify behaviors are predisposing factors, enabling factors, and reinforcing factors. **Predisposing factors** consist of an individual's knowledge and traits such as attitudes, beliefs, values, and perceptions. **Enabling factors** consist of access to healthcare facilities, services, resources, providers, and transportation. **Reinforcing factors** involve rewards and feedback after the behavior change has occurred. Family, friends, and teachers can use reinforcing factors, such as recognition, appreciation, admiration (Green & Kreuter, 2005).

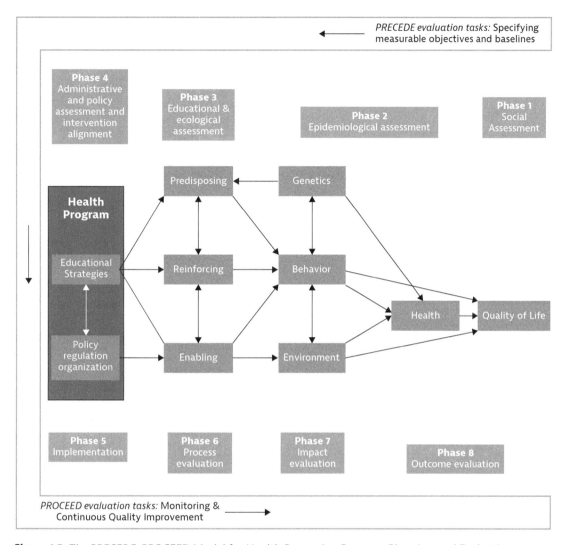

Figure 6.7 *The PRECEDE-PROCEED Model for Health Promotion Program Planning and Evaluation.*

Phase 4 is known as *administrative policy assessment* and *intervention alignment. Admin-istrative policy* planners identify if there are enough resources available for the planned intervention.

Phases 5–8 make up the PROCEED section of the model, when implementation and evaluation of the planned intervention take place. Phase 5 is known as *implementation,* when strategies and resources are chosen and the implementation of the intervention takes place. Phases 6–8 consist of *process, impact,* and *outcome evaluation,* when objectives are outlined in the assessment process.

Summary

This chapter explored various health education and health promotion theories that have evolved from a variety of different disciplines. This chapter provides an overview of some of the critical theories used in our discipline. You have been introduced to key terms such as theory, model, concept, construct, and variables, which are crucial in understanding how to apply theories in different situations and settings. A central role of health educators is to plan, implement, and evaluate programs and behaviors. Each of the theories and models presented in this chapter can aid in the design of effective interventions for individuals and communities.

Review Questions

1. Explain the difference between constructs and variables.

2. Explain what a stage theory is and how it differs from continuum theory.

3. What five intervention areas should the socio-ecological model assess?

4. Explain the six original constructs associated with the health belief model.

5. State and define the seven areas of the transtheoretical model of behavior change.

6. Define social cognitive theory and list five examples of specific constructs associated with this theory.

7. Explain the various levels of the diffusion of innovation theory of behavior change.

8. Explain the difference between the two planning models in health promotion.

Case Scenario

You have been elected the new student president at your university. Your first role of business is to decrease the rate of drug overdoses on your campus. After reviewing the various health promotion theories presented to you by the wellness educator on campus, which theory would you suggest the campus adopt to plan and implement an effective program? Plan out each step or construct of the theory as if you were going to implement it.

Critical Thinking Questions

1. In your own life, think of a situation/circumstance that you wanted to change. For example, maybe you tried to stop smoking. What behavior change model would you implement? Plan out the stages/constructs. What outcome(s) are you looking for to determine effectiveness?

2. You are working in a health club as a personal trainer, and you see a new member walk in to sign up for a membership. After speaking with her, you learn she needs to lose 100 pounds. She states she has been on many fad diets but never sticks with them. She has

never liked exercise but knows it will help her with her weight loss goals. She is ready to make a change today. What level of the transtheoretical model of behavior change is the new member at? What steps must she take to get to the last stage of this model—termination? What would you change if she "relapsed?"

3. Recreate the diffusion of innovation curve (Figure 6.4) with your family or friends. Think of the smartphone or any piece of smart technology. Who are the early adopters in your family, and who are the early majority, the late majority, and the laggards? Explain why each member is at each phase of the diffusion of innovation theory.

Activity

After reviewing Chapter 6, you should be familiar with the several different models and theories used in this profession. You will now be asked to apply the knowledge from these theoretical frameworks into your behavior change intervention. A friend who needs your help in quitting smoking has approached you. You have decided to use your knowledge from Chapter 6 to guide you in creating a reliable and effective intervention for your friend.

- Choose the planning model or theory you think would best fit your friend in her pursuits to quit smoking. Identify this theory or model and how you would explain to her how you will use it to help her change her behavior.

- Describe the history of the model/theory. Use this chapter and reputable outside sources to find the history behind the theory/model.

Web Links

http://ctb.ku.edu/en/4-developing-framework-or-model-change

Community Toolbox

At this website, developing frameworks for models of change are introduced. This website can aid you in the chapter activity assignment at the end of the chapter.

https://www.healthypeople.gov/2020/tools-and-resources/program-planning/implement

Healthy People 2020

This website uses links, tools, and strategies to help communities reach health goals. You can use this website for data or to develop a framework or model for change.

http://people.umass.edu/aizen/tpb.html

Theory of Planned Behavior

This website is by Icek Ajzen, the creator of the theory of planned behavior. This website describes the theory of planned behavior and how to design an intervention using the model.

https://cancercontrol.cancer.gov/brp/research/theories_project/theory.pdf

The Theory at a Glance: A Guide for Health Promotion Practice

The National Cancer Institute created a primer, *Theory at a Glance: A Guide for Health Promotion Practice*. This primer explains thorough descriptions of various models mentioned in this text. It is an excellent supplemental book for understanding the importance of theory.

http://web.uri.edu/cprc/about-ttm/

The Transtheoretical Model

The University of Rhode Island's Cancer Prevention Research Center describes the Transtheoretical Model with a detailed overview and how to measure in each stage of the model.

References

Ajzen, I. (2006). *Theory of planned behavior*. Retrieved from http://www.people.umass.edu/aizen/tpb.html

Bandura, A. (1986). *Social foundations of thought and action*. Englewood Cliffs, NJ: Prentice Hall.

Bandura, A. (2001). Social cognitive theory: An agentic perspective. *Annual Review of Psychology, 52*, 1–26.

Becker, M., Drachman, R., & Kirscht, J. (1974). A new approach to explaining sick-role behavior in low-income populations. *American Journal of Public Health, 64*(3), 205–216.

Burke, N. J., Joseph, G., Pasick, R. J., & Barker, J. C. (2009). Theorizing social context: Rethinking behavioral theory. *Health Education & Behavior, 36* (Suppl. 1), 55S–70S.

Chaplin, J. P., & Krawiec, T. S. (1979). *Systems and theories of psychology* (4th ed.). New York: Holt, Rinehart & Winston.

Cottrell, R., Girvan, J., McKenzie, J., & Seabert, D. (2013). *Principles and Foundations of Health Promotion and Education* (5th ed.). New York: Pearson.

Cottrell, R., Girvan, J., McKenzie, J., & Seabert, D. (2015). *Principles and Foundations of Health Promotion and Education* (6th ed.). New York: Pearson.

Crosby, R. A., Kegler, M. C., & DiClemente, R. J. (2009). Theory in health promotion practice and research. In R. J. DiClemente, R. A. Crosby, & M. C. Kegler (Eds.), *Emerging theories in health promotion practice and research* (2nd ed., pp. 4–17). San Francisco: Jossey-Bass.

Derryberry, M. (2004). Today's health problems and health education. *American Journal of Public Health, 94*(3), 368–371.

Edwards, R. W., Jumper-Thurman, P., Plested, B. A., Oetting, E. R., & Swanson, L. (2000). Community readiness: Research to practice. *Journal of Community Psychology, 28*(3), 291–307.

Glanz, K., Rimer, B. K., & Viswanath, K. (Eds.). (2008). *Health behavior and health education: Theory, research, and practice* (4th ed.). San Francisco: Jossey-Bass.

Green, L. W., & Kreuter, M. W. (2005). *Health promotion program planning: An educational and ecological approach* (4th ed.). Boston, MA: McGraw-Hill.

Hochbaum, G. M. (1958). Public participation in medical screening programs: A socio-psychological study. *Public Health Service Publication, No. 572.* Washington, DC: Government Printing Office.

Janz, N., & Becker, M. (1984). The health belief model: A decade later. *Health Education Quarterly, 11*(1), 1–47. doi: 10.1177/109019818401100101

Keida, E. (2016). Relationship between college students' knowledge of the risk factors for type II diabetes and health behaviors. *Education Doctoral.* Paper 278.

Kegeles, S., Kirscht, J., Haefner, D., & Rosenstock, I. (1965). Survey of beliefs about cancer detection and taking Papanicolaou tests. *Public Health Reports 80(9)*, 815–823.

LaMorte, W. (2019). *The social cognitive theory.* Retrieved from http://sphweb.bumc.bu.edu/otlt/MPH-Modules/SB/BehavioralChangeTheories/BehavioralChangeTheories5.html

McLeroy, K. R., Steckler, A., Goodman, R., & Burdine, J. N. (1992). Health education research, theory, and practice: Future directions. *Health Education Research, Theory, and Practice, 7*(1), 1–8.

McKenzie, J. F., Neiger, B. L., & Thackeray, R. (2013). *Planning, implementing, & evaluating health promotion programs: A primer* (6th edition). New York: Pearson.

Minelli, M. J., & Breckon, D. J. (2009). *Community health education: Settings, roles, and skills* (5th ed.). Sudbury, MA: Jones & Bartlett.

Parcel, G. S., Simons-Morton, B. G., Ohara, N. M., Baranowski, T., Kolbe, L. J., & Bee, D. E. (1987). School promotion of healthful diet and exercise behavior: An integration of organizational change and social learning theory interventions. *Journal of School Health, 57*(4), 150–156. doi:10.1111/j.1746-1561.1987.tb04163.x

Prochaska, J. O. (1979). *Systems of psychotherapy: A transtheoretical analysis.* Homewood, IL: Dorsey Press.

Prochaska, J. O. & DiClemente, C. C. (1982). Transtheoretical therapy: Toward more integrative model change. *Psychotherapy: Theory, Research and Practice, 19*(3), 276–288.

Prochaska, J. O., & Velicer, W. F. (1997). The transtheoretical model of health behavior change. *The American Journal of Health Promotion,12*(1), 38–48.

Rimer, B. K., & Glanz, K. (2005). *Theory at a glance: A guide for health promotion practice* (2nd ed.). (NIH Pub. No. 05-3896). Washington, DC: National Cancer Institute.

Rosenstock, I. (1966). Why people use health services. *Milbank Memorial Fund Quarterly, 44*(2), 366–382. doi: 10.1177/109019818801500203

Rosenstock, I. (1974). Historical origins of the health belief model. *Health Education Behavior, 2*(4), 328–335. doi: 10.1177/109019817400200403

Salazar, L. F., Crosby, R. A., & DiClemente, R. J. (2013). Health behavior in context of the "new" public health. In R. J. DiClemente, L. F. Salazar, & R. A. Crosby, (Eds.), *Health behavior theory for public health: Principles, foundations, and applications* (pp. 3–26). Burlington, MA: Jones & Bartlett Learning.

Credits

CHAPTER 7

Improving and Implementing Health Promotion Through Cultural Competence

Paola Benevento

CHAPTER KEY

<u>Authentic Learning</u>: **using problem-solving of real-life scenarios to explore and discuss content and concepts.**

<u>Knowledge</u>: **the theoretical or practical understanding of a concept.**

<u>Reflection</u>: **contemplation or meditation.**

<u>Practice</u>: **applications of ideas or concepts.**

Chapter Objectives

- **Define** cultural competence and related terminology (*knowledge and reflection*).

- **Characterize** current relationships among cultures regarding health and wellness in the community (*authentic learning, reflection, practice, and collaboration*).

- **Explain** the importance of stakeholders and mobilizing the community (*knowledge and reflection*).

- **Explain** why data collection is such an essential process as it relates to cultural competence and research (*knowledge, reflection, practice, and collaboration*).

- Briefly **describe** the techniques for data collection (*collaboration, practice, and reflection*).

Chapter Links to the Areas of Responsibility of a Health Educator/Health Promotion Professional

- Area of Responsibility I: Assessment and Needs Capacity

- Area of Responsibility II: Planning

- Area of Responsibility V: Advocacy

- Area of Responsibility VII: Communication

Introduction

The core foundation of health promotion centers around group and community aesthetics. It is virtually impossible to begin to think about promoting wellness without thinking about who the intended recipients are. With that being said, one must recognize and value the significant role the community can, and should, play in promoting wellness initiatives. It is important to note that the term "**community**" in this chapter will refer to a **target population** that has formed based on various commonalities rather than solely a geographic one, such as which neighborhood they belong to. Additionally, the individuals who comprise the community or target population will be known as **stakeholders**, individuals who have vested interests in the well-being of the community for various reasons. It is essential to keep in mind that stakeholders play a crucial role in health promotion.

Stakeholders can make your initiative "more responsive to local conditions, while effectively harnessing their knowledge, creativity, and energy to the task" (Razik & Swanson, 2010, p. 300). This chapter will explore the importance of gaining the support of, and mobilizing the community you are working with to improve health conditions as well as strategies that will help you do so.

Importance of Cultural Competence

Any group of people—a school, church, sports team, business, or residents of a neighborhood—come accompanied by their own specific culture. Often when people hear the word "culture," they begin to think of something very distant or foreign. Many fail to realize that any collection of individuals have the ability to develop their own culture, whether intentionally or not.

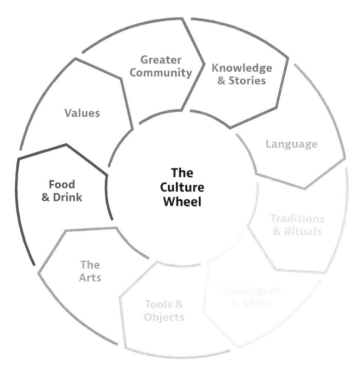

Figure 7.1 *The Culture Wheel.*

According to Haviland, Prins, and Walrath (2016), **"culture"** is a term that refers to the average or typical facets of a group—known as their "shared ideas, values, and perceptions. These are used to make sense of our experiences and generate behavior" (p. 6). This can include but is not limited to language, clothing, food, rituals, behaviors, attitudes, beliefs, and various other social, political, economic, and religious aspects (Haviland, Prins, & Walrath, 2016).

Additionally, any one person can be a part of multiple cultural systems. It is possible, and not uncommon, for an individual to belong to a culture within their family, workplace, neighborhood, and additional groups whose scale can range from being relatively small and more intimate, such as a local community grassroots organization, to a larger size, such as a country. It is essential to recognize not only the importance of the complexities that can exist within each one, but also how they may intertwine with one another. Therefore, it is essential to keep in mind that while you are working with one specific community and their culture, individuals within that community may be bringing with them additional cultural values that could impact your work as a health promotion specialist.

Involving All Stakeholders in the Process

You may have noticed that throughout this chapter, the phrase "working with" has been used repeatedly. It has been used purposefully to emphasize that the stakeholders within the community should be viewed as partners. As previously stated, part of having a positive relationship means having two-way communication and taking the time to not only inform stakeholders but also to listen to what it is that they have to say. DuFour, DuFour, and Eaker (2008) discuss promoting a sense of empowerment and ownership amongst stakeholders as a means of getting everyone involved and on board. They state, "People invest themselves in what they help create" (p. 326). Therefore, if you want your health promotion initiative to be successful, you must engage them as "equal partners" who are involved and contributing. While the target population may not have training in the field of health promotion, they do possess expertise in their community, which will ultimately benefit the process of successfully implementing a program.

Stakeholders should be involved in every part of the process, covering all Eight Areas of Responsibility as described by the National Commission for Health Education Credentialing (2020):

- Area I: Assessment of Needs and Capacity

- Area II: Planning

- Area III: Implementation

- Area IV: Evaluation and Research

- Area V: Advocacy

- Area VI: Communication

- Area VII: Leadership and Management

- Area VIII: Ethics and Professionalism

During your journey through these seven areas, you should be actively looking for ways to involve community members. With that being said, the roles of stakeholders will vary as you move from one area to the next. For example, there will be times when you involve community members by seeking their input as you collect data for a needs assessment (see **Figure 7.2**). At this time, the community can provide you with information concerning their wants, needs, daily practices, and culture, among other things. You may find you have identified several areas of concerns during a needs assessment, and stakeholders can be particularly helpful in working with you to prioritize which are the most important based on their experiences as members of the community. Moving forward in the field of health promotion, you will notice community members can contribute in additional ways. Stakeholders' roles during planning health promotion (Area II) and implementing health promotion (Area III) require them to be more engaged and mobile. Stakeholders transition from being providers of data to partnering with the health promotion specialist(s) to plan and implement the program.

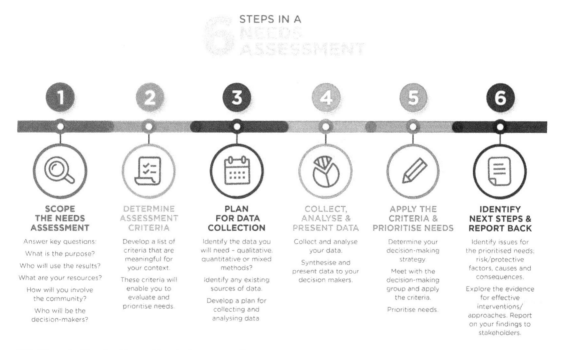

Figure 7.2 *Steps in Conducting a Needs Assessment.*

Since every target population is unique in various respects, the process and program should be equally unique. It is important to remember that a program you use with one community may not apply or be effective within another community, even if the health concerns are similar. Ultimately, by actively and consistently involving the community throughout the Eight Areas of Responsibility, you can create a health promotion program that is tailored to the community you are working with.

Acquiring Cultural Competence

Many anthropologists, specifically cultural anthropologists, have spent their time living amongst the groups they are studying and, in some cases, have even immersed themselves in the groups' day-to-day activities. This practice is a way of working toward becoming **culturally competent** about a targeted group. Betancourt, Green, Carrillo, and Ananeh-Firempong (2003) describe a culturally competent system "as one that acknowledges and incorporates the importance of culture, cross-cultural relations, vigilance toward cultural differences, expansion of cultural knowledge, and adaptation of services to meet culturally unique needs" (p. 294). It is understood that it is not always realistic for someone to move their place of residency and physically live within the community they are working with. Instead, the point to be emphasized is that knowing the target population you are working with and genuinely becoming competent in their culture is essential for the successful implementation of your health program. There are other effective ways of doing so, such as immersing yourself in the social structure, interviewing members of the target population, surveying the target population, conducting focus groups, direct observation, etc.

Again, these tactics of gaining an understanding of your target population do not refer to merely a surface-level understanding. Instead, if health promotion specialists wish to be able to achieve a deep level of knowledge beyond the superficial, it requires them to engage with three main components: commitment, physical immersion, and open-mindedness. Being **committed** to an initiative means dedicating your time and efforts to learning about and bringing about change, with the understanding that projects may stray from expected timelines due to the unique specificities different communities possess. **Physical immersion** refers to the health promotion specialists spending time within the physical boundaries the target population occupies, including physical interactions with individuals of the community within these spaces. Lastly, **open-mindedness** means understanding that the communities and individuals you are working with will possess perspectives that differ from your own. It entails being able to value their attitudes and beliefs in addition to your own and going into the community free of preconceived notions/biases.

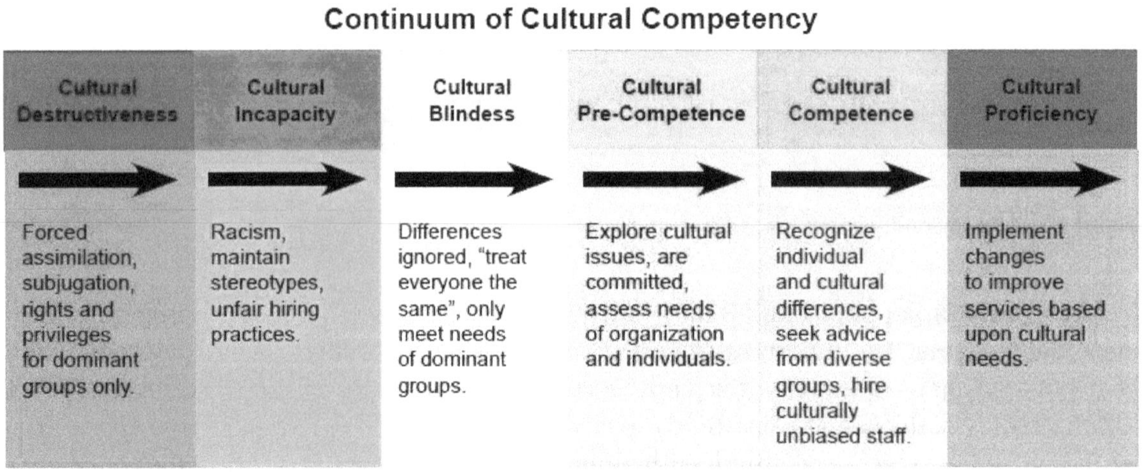

Continuum of Cultural Competency

Cultural Destructiveness	Cultural Incapacity	Cultural Blindess	Cultural Pre-Competence	Cultural Competence	Cultural Proficiency
Forced assimilation, subjugation, rights and privileges for dominant groups only.	Racism, maintain stereotypes, unfair hiring practices.	Differences ignored, "treat everyone the same", only meet needs of dominant groups.	Explore cultural issues, are committed, assess needs of organization and individuals.	Recognize individual and cultural differences, seek advice from diverse groups, hire culturally unbiased staff.	Implement changes to improve services based upon cultural needs.

Figure 7.3 *The Continuum of Cultural Competence for Health Educators.*

Ensuring Cultural Competence in Data Collection

Cultural competence requires thorough data collection to gain a holistic view. Two widely recognized forms of data to consider are *quantitative* and *qualitative*. Quantitative data refers to information that has to do primarily with numbers and statistics. According to the Centers for Disease Control and Prevention, it is a type of collection that works to "generate numerical data such as frequencies, percentages or rates" (Centers for Disease Control and Prevention, 2010)—for example, information you would pull from a census, such as percentages of ethnic groups within a population, median household incomes, employment rates, education rates, and percentages of individuals with or without health insurance coverage. This data is useful because it can provide you with a starting point in terms of gaining background information, in addition to helping identify patterns and trends within the community. This is an excellent place to start before you move to the *physical immersion* stage so you can have a baseline understanding of the target population you will be working with and make the most of your time when you do interact in this setting.

Quantitative data can also resurface in latter parts of the process, depending on what you discover and how you wish to use it, such as to evaluate the program for effectiveness. While quantitative data aids in understanding *what* is happening, qualitative data works to explain *why* it is happening. The Centers for Disease Control and Prevention describe qualitative methods as "those that produce descriptive information" and that "add depth, detail, and meaning to your research" (Centers for Disease Control and Prevention, 2010). Often, people associate qualitative data collection with the humanities and social sciences because it is an interactive process between human beings. However, you will find that regardless of the field of study, whenever a human component is present, there is an insight to be gained from employing qualitative practices.

As previously stated, you can use quantitative data findings to guide your questioning and areas of focus for the qualitative component. For example, if you learn the median annual income in a neighborhood is $22,000, during the qualitative phase, you may wish to design several questions around employment and finances if you see them as relevant to promoting your health initiative within the community.

Participating in data collection not only helps with collecting information relevant to the needs assessment portion of the process, but it also helps the health promotion specialist learn about the culture of the community and how the two are intertwined. For example, if it is identified that an elementary school has a health concern around children being overweight and you learn a cultural norm for that neighborhood is to purchase affordable but unhealthy snacks at the local bodega, you can begin to see a link between the two. Understanding the behaviors, beliefs, attitudes, and patterns that primarily contribute to the culture is necessary when working to institute a successful action plan.

Creating Positive Relationships

A foundational element that will work to increase your chances of successfully implementing health initiatives is establishing a positive relationship with your target population that

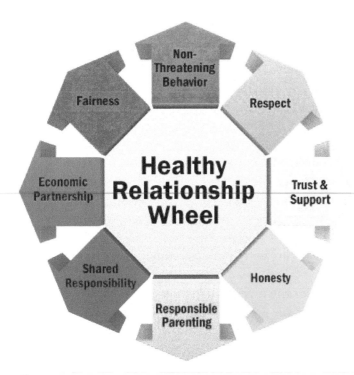

Figure 7.4 *Building Healthy Relationships.*

consists of mutual respect and trust. Moran (2004) claims "the absence of trust impedes effectiveness and progress" (p. 41). This is especially important for the field of health promotion because, ultimately, the goal is to make effective progress toward a meaningful change. Failing to establish and maintain positive relationships can create unnecessary obstacles that may slow down, lessen the significance, or even lead to the demise of your initiative. Developing respect and trust between the community and health promotion specialists is not something that can happen instantly (see **Figure 7.4**). These are states of being that you have to put a conscious and consistent effort towards.

To help foster this type of relationship, individuals within the target population must know not only that you are there with good intentions but also that you have a strong commitment to them and their health. As stated previously that commitment, physical immersion, and open-mindedness were deemed necessary to becoming culturally competent, they are equally essential when working with community members to build solid relationships. The phrase *"talking the talk* versus *walking the walk"* applies to this concept. It is easy to say you are invested in a community, but you must show your commitment by spending time with stakeholders in their community and being open to the knowledge there is to be gained.

During the needs assessment phase, you may learn that you possess different cultural norms and therefore view things differently than the target population you are working with. However, when entering a community, you must do so with respect for the individuals and their culture. It is unreasonable to believe you will be in agreeance with all the perspectives, beliefs, and behaviors you come across in your work. Still, you must understand that you are not there to judge or criticize but to promote practices that encourage a healthier state for the members of the community. Part of demonstrating respect is treating stakeholders like humans and not subjects. Always being reflective of the work you do and how your actions may affect the everyday lives of community members shows you have high regard for their wellbeing. After all, the community and culture that stakeholders are members of, are not something they can easily walk away from.

When beginning your work with a community, you must acknowledge past relationships and how they may impact your current one. Often the struggles stakeholders are facing are not new, and with that in mind, there may have been failed past efforts. Leaving when things do not go as planned or making promises that have no follow-through are ways to hinder the building of trust in the present and the future. Therefore, when setting goals for your initiative, you want to be realistic so you are not promoting false hopes within a community. It is okay to start with a small goal and then build a larger and more long-term goal. Setting and attaining small-scale goals is an excellent way to establish trust because it demonstrates a dedication to stakeholders.

A key contributor to trust, respect, and building an overall strong relationship is communication. Communication refers to the exchange of ideas between two parties. There must be a consistent flow of information, not only from the health promotion specialists to the target population but also from the target population to the health promotion specialists. When a strong sense of trust is present in a relationship, communication flows more freely (Moran, 2004). This helps ensure both parties are fully equipped with the information necessary to breed success. When both parties can communicate with each other, it also strengthens the relationship because everyone involved can feel like equal contributors.

Summary

What is health promotion? It is *chang*ing. It is identifying a specific health-related concern amongst a target population and working with them to change behavior and patterns to positively impact their health. Change is a concept that gets talked about in various respects: some people fear it, while some people desire it. When working with a targeted demographic, the last thing you want to do is have stakeholders fear change or push back against it.

This chapter discussed ways you can combat pushback and work to get stakeholders in your target population both supporting and participating in your health initiative as you move towards change. Manley and Hawkins (2010) state that we must be aware and have sensitivity toward issues that relate to beliefs and culture.

If you are serious about implementing meaningful long-term change within a target population, you must take the time to get to know the culture and work to build strong positive relationships with open communication. Most importantly, we must be open to the value the community and its stakeholders possess.

Review Questions

1. According to the reading, what does it mean to be "culturally competent"?

2. What are the three main components a health promotion specialist should be knowledgeable in to develop a deep understanding of a specific culture?

3. How might collecting data on a specific culture help you increase your cultural competence?

4. What characteristics must a health promotion specialist possess to build proper trust and respect for a specific culture?

Case Scenario

The Orange community is a neighborhood on the south side of a large urban city. This community is one of the most impoverished in the city, with high unemployment rates, struggling businesses with rapid turnover, access to unreliable public transportation, limited private/personal transportation, and most residents possessing a high school/equivalent degree or less.

This neighborhood has been labeled a "food desert" by local activists and community members, which refers to areas that lack access to healthy and affordable foods. Within the neighborhood, food options consist of fast-food chains, several locally owned restaurants, and corner stores roughly every two to three blocks. The nearest grocery store is located 2.5 miles away, and the nearest bulk grocery store is 7 miles away.

After meeting with a local community organizer, you learn there have been several past initiatives that have failed. One failed initiative aimed to address two issues (the community being a food desert and a lack of physical activity) by organizing walking trips to the nearest grocery store. Due to the high number of individuals who were age 60 and above, the plan had a low turnout rate and did not solve the health concerns. This has led to a lack of trust amongst residents and an unwillingness to cooperate with health promotion specialists entering the neighborhood. During your meeting with the local community organizer, she did note that a large percentage of the target population attend worship services and go to events at the local community center together.

Additionally, the Orange community prides itself on being very close-knit and the fact that stakeholders are committed to helping one another daily. What do you think will be your biggest challenge? How would you utilize stakeholders in your target population to address this challenge? Why do you think the health promotion specialists who organized the community walk failed? What would you have done differently if you had been a part of that team?

Critical Thinking Questions

1. If you are conducting a qualitative research study using semistructured interviews, how will you ensure cultural competence in your data collection processes?

2. Based on the reading from this chapter, what cultural systems are you a part of? How do your cultural systems impact how you build relationships with others?

3. What knowledge and understanding would you need to acquire as a health educator in order to conduct a needs assessment in a community you do not live in and are not familiar with?

Activities

1. Think back on a time from your academic career when you felt included and appreciated for what you were doing. Now think again on a time when you felt excluded or unappreciated. Were there any differences in the way the two different scenarios made you feel? How did it impact your behaviors? What consistencies do you notice in the

situations in which people felt excluded? How do you think those experiences can be related to cultural competencies?

2. After watching the TED Talk video *A Danger of a Single Story* (https://www.ted.com/ talks/chimamanda_ngozi_adichie_the_danger_of_a_single_story?language=en), what resonates with you? How can we find our cultural voice? What takeaways are essential for you to note as a health educator who will implement health promotion programs in the community?

3. Think about your multicultural self and how we build positive relationships with others. Place your name in the center of a circle. Write an essential aspect of your identity in four circles that branch out from your center circle. Each small circle should represent an identifier or descriptor you feel is critical in defining you. This can include anything: Asian American, female, mother, athlete, educator, Catholic, or any descriptor with which you identify. Partner with someone in the class and share a story about a time when you were proud to be recognized with one of the descriptors you identified in your circles. After the discussion, share a story about a time when it was especially painful to identify with one of your identifiers.

Web Links

https://www.nchec.org/responsibilities-and-competencies

Responsibilities and Competencies of a Health Educator

This website outlines the areas of responsibilities for a health educator.

https://www.samhsa.gov/section-223/cultural-competence

CCBHCs and Cultural Competence

This website outlines the general requirements of cultural competence as well as training and care.

https://www.ncbi.nlm.nih.gov/pmc/articles/PMC1803701/

The Case for Cultural Competence in Health Professions Education

This journal article discusses how we are addressing cultural competence in the U.S. curricula in higher academia.

https://www.ted.com/talks/chimamanda_ngozi_adichie_the_danger_of_a_single_story?language=en

The Danger of a Single Story

Chimamanda Ngozi Adichie describes how our cultures and lives are composed of many overlapping stories.

References

Betancourt, J. R., Green, A. R., Carrillo, E., & Ananeh-Firempong II, O. (2003). *Defining cultural competence: A practical framework for addressing racial/ethnic disparities in health and health care. Public Health Reports, 118,* p. 294.

Centers for Disease Control and Prevention. (2010, August 9). *Gateway to Health Communication & Social Marketing Practice.* Retrieved from https://www.cdc.gov/healthcommunication/cdcynergy/Evaluation.html

DuFour, R., DuFour, R., & Eaker, R. (2008). *Revisiting professional learning communities at work: new insights for improving schools.* Bloomington, IN: Solution Tree Press.

Fowler, F. J. (2013). *Survey research methods: Applied social research methods (5th ed.). Thousand Oaks, CA:* SAGE Publications.

Grogan, M. (2013). *The Jossey-Bass reader on educational leadership (3rd ed.).* San Francisco, CA: Jossey-Bass.

Guest, G., Namey, E .E., & Mitchell, M. L. (2013). *Collecting qualitative data: A field manual for applied research. Thousand Oaks, CA:* SAGE Publications.

Haviland, W. A., Prins, H., Walrath, D., & McBride, B. (2016). *Cultural anthropology: The human challenge (15th ed.).* Boston, MA: Cengage Learning.

Krueger, R. A., & Casey, M. A. (2015). *Focus groups: A practical guide for applied research (5th ed.). Thousand Oaks, CA:* SAGE Publications.

Manley, R. J., & Hawkins, R. J. (2010). *Designing school systems for all students.* Lanham, MD: Rowman and Littlefield.

National Commission for Health Education Credentialing. (2020). *Responsibilities and competencies for health education specialists.* Retrieved from https://www.nchec.org/responsibilities-and-competencies

Razik, T. A, & Swanson, A. D. (2010). *Fundamental concepts of educational leadership & management.* Boston, MA: Allyn & Bacon.

Taylor, S. J., Bogdan, R., & DeVault, M. (2016). *Introduction to qualitative research methods.* Hoboken, NJ: Wiley & Sons, Inc.

Credits

CHAPTER 8

Achieving Wellness Through Philosophy

CHAPTER KEY

Authentic Learning: **using problem-solving of real-life scenarios to explore and discuss content and concepts.**

Knowledge: **the theoretical or practical understanding of a concept.**

Reflection: **contemplation or meditation.**

Practice: **applications of ideas or concepts.**

Chapter Objectives

Upon completion of this chapter and participating in the critical thinking questions at the end, you should be able to:

- **Define** the terms "philosophy" and "philodox" (*knowledge and reflection*).

- **Discuss** the importance of philosophy in health education and health promotion discipline (*authentic learning, reflection, practice, and collaboration*).

- **Explain** and identify the predominant health promotion philosophies (*knowledge and reflection*).

- **Create** your health and wellness philosophy (*authentic learning, reflection, practice, and collaboration*).

Chapter Links to the Areas of Responsibility of a Health Educator/Health Promotion Professional

- Area of Responsibility I: Assessment and Needs Capacity

- Area of Responsibility II: Planning

- Area of Responsibility V: Advocacy

- Area of Responsibility VI: Communication

- Area of Responsibility VII: Leadership and Management

- Area of Responsibility VIII: Ethics and Professionalism

Introduction

The purpose of discussing health promotion philosophies is to provide health educators with guidance to practice within the profession. When you use a philosophical framework, you can approach various scenarios and situations in different ways. Before you can take action to gain optimal health, you must think about what you believe the essential elements are in health and wellness. Today many of us have beliefs and views on politics and religion, but when it comes to our health, we do not often give it much thought until we are in crisis. As a future health educator, you must think about what you believe are the best approaches to optimizing your health and identifying the key steps to effectively implementing them in your life. In this chapter, you will learn about predominant health philosophies, how having a philosophy can impact your delivery of health promotion, and how to write your health philosophy.

Philosophy

The term "**philosophy**" literally means "love of wisdom" and is the study of knowledge, or "thinking about thinking." Philosophy is a discipline concerned with questions about how we should live, work, and play (ethics), the nature of reality and being (metaphysics), genuine knowledge (epistemology), and principles of reasoning (logic). Philosophy, a term initially used by ancient Greeks, is done primarily through reflection and does not tend to rely on experiments. It provides a way of thinking about a wide range of issues and gives a method to analyze arguments that can be useful in a variety of life situations. A philosophy, in the broad sense, encompasses one's attitudes, values, principles, and beliefs. As human beings, we all have convictions, ideas, values, experiences, and opinions about different areas that apply to life; these are the building blocks that make up one's philosophy.

In the field of health education and health promotion, high-order questions are essential for both practitioners and researchers to think about when establishing a health philosophy. We must start by taking a systematic look at some fundamental questions:

- Why do we need good health?

- Why is it important to be healthy?

- Who are we?

- What areas of the human condition do we choose to affect?
- Why do we do the things we do?
- Why do we do things in the manner we do?
- What difference are they making?

Health education specialists should promote diverse ideas and encourage critical thinking (Gambescia, 2013). A life shaped by **philodox**, which is known as the "love of one's own opinion," can impede a health educator's ability to contribute to the health of all people. The philodox approach is used by someone who is more argumentative, rejects the possibility of any other alternative explanation, and lets opinion define their reality. Philodox hinders the discovery of new knowledge, facts, or insight into the field of health education and health promotion. Without a philosophy, individuals may start to use opinion over fact. As health educators, we must use philosophy to help explain an issue so true meaning can form. Today you see philosophies everywhere. Individuals have their philosophies that incorporate their attitudes, principles, beliefs, values, and concepts. You also see groups, organizations, and companies that have philosophies, which are known as **mission statements**.

> Individual = philosophy statement
> Group = mission statement

A mission statement is considered a philosophical position that conveys an organization's values or beliefs. For instance, the American Cancer Society's mission statement is to "save lives, celebrate lives, and lead the fight for a world without cancer" (American Cancer Society, 2017). After reading this statement, it is clear that this organization is dedicated to the health and welfare of the public through prevention and treatment. Often, many health educators will read organizations' mission statements before applying for positions to make sure their philosophy, values, and beliefs are represented and align with that company or organization. Corporations also have their philosophical positions or slogans that can be trying to sell a product or service. For instance, take some of the most well-known company phrases, such as "Just Do It" by Nike or "Think Different" by Apple. The use of catchy phrases like these is meant to show their interest in the people. If the public believes these phrases are true representations of the companies' values, they are more likely to buy or use their services and products.

A person's philosophy is also seen in quotes and sayings. For instance, think back to your senior year in high school. Were you asked to have a senior quote in the yearbook? Did you choose a quote that embodied your attitude, values, and beliefs? Did you select a quote that represents your personality? The American activist Sam Berns, who suffered from a rare disease known as progeria, had a three-part philosophy of life at the age of 17. Berns (2013) stated: "(1) Be okay with what you ultimately can't do because there is so much you *can* do; (2) surround yourself with people you want to be around; and (3) keep moving forward" (Berns, 2014). A philosophy is rarely stagnant. It is often continuous, showing what is essential within the world and how to move forward with a positive outlook on life. One of the most influential health education specialists in our discipline has noted that philosophy does not have to be abstract. It allows people to integrate their past, present, and future through a framework that guides them through life (Bensley, 1993).

The Importance of a Personal Philosophy for Health Educators

Why create a philosophy? Today we are often told who we should be. It is essential to know how to forge our paths and define our successes and values. Having a philosophy helps guide us through the complex world of life. A philosophy helps form a basis of reality and is a part of our growth as human beings. As you grow older, you encounter new experiences and gain new insights, and you may find that your philosophy of life changes. This is normal and can often be an endless task.

Figure 8.1 *Dr. Joycelyn Elders, the first African American appointed Surgeon General.*

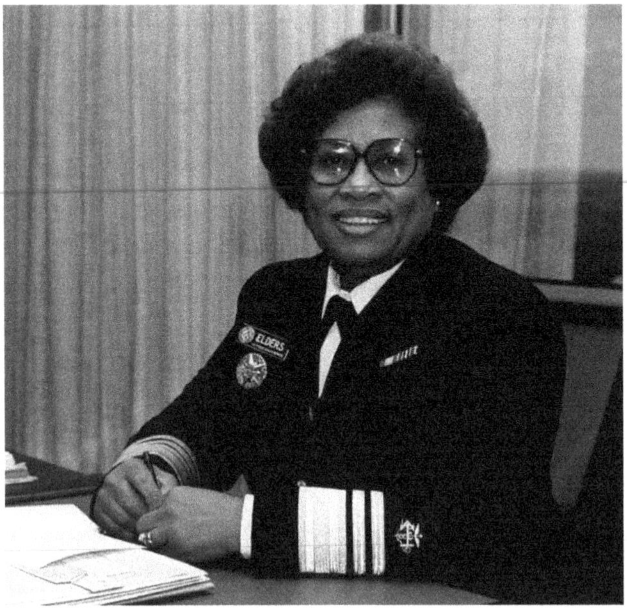

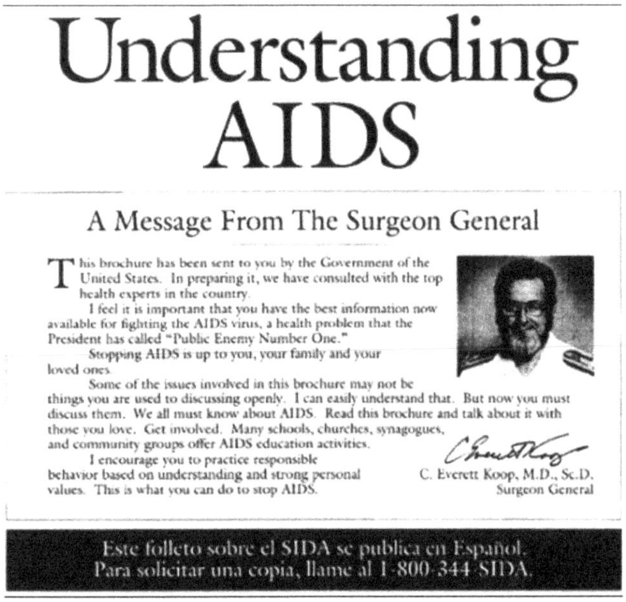

Understanding AIDS

A Message From The Surgeon General

This brochure has been sent to you by the Government of the United States. In preparing it, we have consulted with the top health experts in the country.

I feel it is important that you have the best information now available for fighting the AIDS virus, a health problem that the President has called "Public Enemy Number One."

Stopping AIDS is up to you, your family and your loved ones.

Some of the issues involved in this brochure may not be things you are used to discussing openly. I can easily understand that. But now you must discuss them. We all must know about AIDS. Read this brochure and talk about it with those you love. Get involved. Many schools, churches, synagogues, and community groups offer AIDS education activities.

I encourage you to practice responsible behavior based on understanding and strong personal values. This is what you can do to stop AIDS.

C. Everett Koop, M.D., Sc.D.
Surgeon General

Este folleto sobre el SIDA se publica en Español.
Para solicitar una copia, llame al 1-800-344-SIDA.

Figure 8.2 *C. Everett Coop, the 13th Surgeon General of the United States.*

It is essential for health educators to have personal philosophies because the profession of health education is considered a helping profession, and those who work in this profession should value helping others. Having your philosophy provides a framework for how you consistently act toward other people and often reflects the importance of people in general. As health educators, our primary concern is to protect, prevent, empower, and advocate for health and wellness. To do this, we must have a philosophy that aligns with our discipline. However, one might hold many philosophies. You may see individuals who have their philosophies of life and their opinions of health education. Having multiple philosophies just guides you in how you live, work, and play.

A well-reasoned philosophy often plays a vital role in your career path. There are some notable instances where health educators' philosophies clashed with their career roles, posing moral and ethical dilemmas. Take Joycelyn Elders, for example. Appointed by President Bill Clinton in 1993, Dr. Elders became the first African American to serve as Surgeon General of the United States. Her outspoken views about reproductive rights outraged the religious right. She favored handing out condoms to public school children to prevent teen pregnancy and promote safe sex (Schonfeld, 2016). Ultimately, her philosophy sparked controversy, and conservative outrage erupted, leading to her resignation in 1994.

Another scenario where personal philosophy impacted someone's career involved United States Surgeon General C. Everett Koop, who was confronted with the AIDS epidemic during his career. Koop was a staunch conservative Christian leader who was against drug use and premarital sex. However, Koop was in favor of HIV/AIDS education, stressing that the epidemic was a health crisis that required preventative education. This further illustrates the impact of philosophy on our profession. From both examples, we see how these individuals' philosophies had the primary concern of protecting and enhancing the health of those they served.

Philosophies Associated with Health and Wellness

In Chapter 1, we discussed the progression of health promotion and wellness through understanding of key health terminology. In Chapter 2, we discussed the importance of the eight wellness dimensions. This understanding will help build upon several predominant health philosophies that we use in our profession.

Health educators encourage balance, otherwise known as symmetry. **The philosophy of symmetry** consists of four of the eight wellness dimensions: physical, emotional, spiritual, and social wellness components. The philosophy of symmetry explains that each of these wellness components has the same importance and should be balanced equally. Rash (1985) believes that good health begins with a richness and enjoyment of life that makes individuals help others more willingly. Those who seek to enhance the health of others and serve others should embody a philosophy of symmetry (Rash, 1985).

Another philosophical framework that focuses on balance is the **holistic health philosophy**. This philosophy achieves health and quality of life by balancing three modalities—mind, body, and spirit—for a whole being. In addition to balancing, individuals with this framework focus on learning new and natural forms of well-being and healing so others can experience long-lasting healing and well-being. This holistic view of health gives one a renewed sense of personal fulfillment and purpose in life.

The **wellness philosophy** looks at balancing all eight of the wellness dimensions to form a "healthy person." Those who believe in a wellness philosophy state that

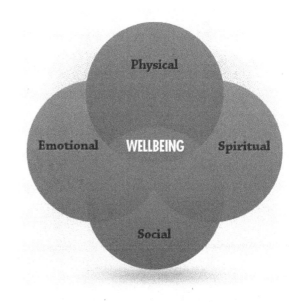

Figure 8.3 *The Philosophy of Symmetry.*

all people can achieve some wellness, no matter what their obstacles are. From previous chapters, we know that health and wellness is not just the absence of disease or illness: it is a dynamic state of awareness and self-empowerment that enhances our essence as human beings.

You may follow one or more of the philosophies above in how you live, work, and play. Each of these philosophies can help you develop your opinion about health and how it would apply to your career path. Health educators need to distinguish what they value in their own lives and also in their health. By understanding these key components, you will be better suited to help others create their philosophies of health and what is important to them in their lives. In addition to these philosophies, there are five other predominant health philosophies that health educators use on a day-to-day basis when working with patients, clients, organizations, students, etc.

Predominant Health Philosophies

Welle, Russell, and Kittleson (1995) conducted research to determine if health educators used any specific philosophies in their work. It was determined that there are five predominant health philosophies that health educators use: behavior change philosophy, cognitive-based philosophy, decision-making philosophy, freeing or functioning philosophy, and social change philosophy.

The behavior change philosophy involves the use of behavior change contracts, goal set-ting, and self-monitoring to help clients or individuals foster healthy habits. This philosophy uses **s**pecific, **m**easurable, **a**chievable, **r**ealistic, and **t**imely **(SMART) goals/objectives** to help individuals set small goals that are realistic and can help aid in the modification of unhealthy habits. As a health educator, you may use this philosophy when working with clients who are trying to quit smoking, increase physical activity, decrease stress, get more sleep, etc. For exam-ple, a health educator might have a client who wants to lose weight. When meeting with the client or patient, you may create goals for the individual to help with their weight loss process. Ensuring the goals/objectives are SMART will increase the likelihood that the client/patient knows exactly what they need to do to achieve their goal(s). This would embody the behavior change philosophy.

The cognitive-based philosophy focuses on content and factual information. By using content and factual information, you can increase the knowledge of individuals to make better choices. As a health educator, you may use this philosophy when working with a patient or client who is unaware of the risk of a disease or illness. For example, if you have a client who is engaging in risky sexual behavior and does not believe they are susceptible to HIV/AIDS, you may want to use the cognitive-based philosophy. You would want to educate this client and show mortality statistics and facts so they are aware of their susceptibility to the virus.

The decision-making philosophy uses cases or scenarios to help individuals analyze potential solutions and develop skills to approach health-related decisions. This philosophy has a partic-ular emphasis on thinking and lifelong learning and is preferred by health education specialists. This philosophy allows an individual to have the tools and skills to make well-informed health decisions in the future: for example, posing different questions about a scenario, such as "What are the alternatives? What is uncertainty? Are there high-risk consequences?" You can help work that problem out and give the individual the tools to understand the best approaches or decisions. Therefore, when they are faced with situations in the future, they will have the skills to work through the event successfully.

The freeing and functioning philosophy was created by Greenberg (1978) and added a critical concept to the decision-making philosophy. This philosophy uses the same ideas from the decision-making philosophy but makes it clear that the individual is free to make their own decision, ultimately freeing individuals to make the best possible choices based on their own needs and interests: for example, giving a client a scenario about drinking and driving, working through the potential risks, and then allowing the client the opportunity to make their own decisions related to alcohol.

The social change philosophy looks at creating social and political change that benefits the health of an individual, group, or community. Health education specialists who embody this philosophy are often on the front lines of creating laws, policies, and ordinances related to health and wellness. For example, a health educator may petition for smoke-free parks as a means to create a healthier environment for communities.

Another interesting finding from Welle, Russell, and Kittleson's (1995) research was the identification of the **eclectic health education/promotion philosophy**. This philosophy simply identifies that health educators are resourceful and adaptable and use many different types of philosophies when working in the field. Sometimes we are using more than one philosophy at a time, making it eclectic. It is not unusual to see a health educator using both the behavior change philosophy and the cognitive-based philosophy to address issues with one individual. It is time to think about what values and beliefs you have when it comes to health and also when it comes to working with clients and patients. How do you see yourself using each of these philosophies?

Each of these philosophies is used to guide health educators when working in the field. They provide a framework and mindset to aid in prevention, promotion, empowerment, and **advocacy** surrounding the health of individuals and communities.

Developing Your Own Health Philosophy

Now that you understand how vital philosophy is, not just in your own life but within the profession of health education and promotion, it is time to explore ways in which you can create your own. You should start brainstorming about the following to compose a philosophy statement:

1. What does a health educator do? What is important to health educators?

2. Construct a list of your values and beliefs.

3. What does health mean to you?

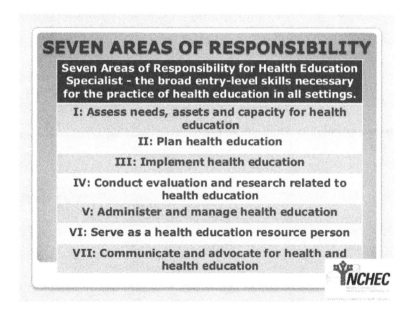

Figure 8.4 *Areas of Responsibility for a Health Educator.*

4. What are some attributes of people you admire and trust?

5. Can you think of some results of studies, meaningful readings, or quotes that impacted you?

6. What are some outcomes you would like to see from health education in the future?

First, you want to think about what a health educator does and what is important to us. Think about the responsibilities of a health educator and how those impact your health philosophy.

What areas of responsibility do you value as a health educator? What responsibilities and values are most important to include in your philosophy? The seven areas of responsibility for a health educator are critical in our profession, and they show dedication to excellence in the practice of promoting individual, family, organizational, and community health (NCHEC, 2019).

Secondly, in drafting your philosophy, you want to start to construct a list of both your values and beliefs. Use **Figure 8.5** to help you create your list.

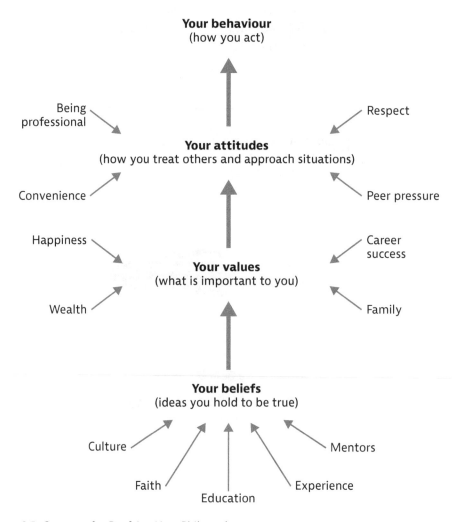

Figure 8.5 *Concepts for Drafting Your Philosophy.*

After you have constructed your list of personal values and beliefs, start thinking about what health means to you personally. Write out a sentence or two that explains what health means to you. Then you want to think about people in your life you admire and trust. What did those individuals embody that made you trust them? Why did you respect them? What traits did they have that you believe are important and valuable characteristics? Now start to think about past readings, results of studies, or quotes that have been impactful for you. Why were they meaningful? What about those quotes stuck with you? Lastly, thinking about the future of your career as a health educator, what outcomes would you like to see in health education and health promotion? From this list you have created, go back and look for common themes. Were there similar characteristics? Are there things that seem more important than others? If so, circle these and make sure to include them in your philosophy statement. After exploring why you value the topics represented, you should be able to compose a philosophy statement that embodies how you live, work, and play. Remember, this statement may change over the years as you grow and experience new things and gain new insights. Personal philosophies are unique and can be created in various ways but will ultimately reflect your way of thinking, acting, and viewing the world.

Summary

A philosophy embodies an individual's values, attitudes, beliefs, and ideas. It is used as a guide for how we live, work, and play. Health education specialists use philosophies to aid in addressing health issues impacting individuals and communities. By having a philosophy as a framework, it can guide many significant decisions in our lives and our health. There are many different health and wellness philosophies health educators can adopt: (1) philosophy of symmetry, (2) holistic health philosophy, (3) wellness philosophy, (4) behavior change philosophy, (5) cognitive-based philosophy, (6) decision-making philosophy, (7) freeing-functioning philosophy, (8) social change philosophy, and (9) eclectic health education and health promotion philosophy. By using these philosophical viewpoints, we can better the well-being of individuals and their quality of life.

Review Questions

1. Define philosophy and philodox. Explain how they differ from each other and why.

2. Explain what the philosophies of symmetry, holistic health, and wellness all have in common.

3. As a future health educator, why is it essential to have not only a personal philosophy but also a philosophy of health?

4. How did United States Surgeon Generals Joycelyn Elders's and C. Everett Koop's philosophies impact their careers?

5. Define the following health and wellness philosophies:
   a. Behavior change philosophy
   b. Cognitive-based philosophy
   c. Decision-making philosophy

d. Freeing-functioning philosophy
e. Social change philosophy
f. Eclectic health education and health promotion philosophy

Case Scenario

You are a student at a local university that is considered a smoke-free campus. However, as a senior, you have been on campus for 4 years and have experienced smokers consistently outside of campus buildings. The second-hand smoke and the piles of cigarettes outside the library have you extremely concerned.

You notice a flyer stating the president of the university is going to be doing "drop-in days" when you can go and ask her questions. You decide to attend the event and speak with the president about your concerns regarding the smoke-free campus and the policy surrounding it.

During this conversation, you realize there are no consequences for students on campus who are smoking. The president explains that it is up to members of the campus community to address those who are not abiding by the smoke-free policy. The president agrees with your concerns and asks you to share your philosophy on this topic so she can take it to the administration. Using the steps outlined in this chapter, write your philosophical position on a smoke-free campus. Based on your philosophy statement, explain what predominant health philosophy you are most identifying with from the chapter and explain why. Lastly, what is your advice to both the president and the administration regarding this health issue on campus?

Critical Thinking Questions

1. A client approaches you and states they want to have greater financial wellness. What philosophy would you use to guide you in this process, and why?

2. You work for a local county health department, and you are creating a program geared toward education and awareness of uterine cancer. Your goal is to increase visits for preventive screenings. What type of mission statement would you create?

3. You just graduated from college and received a job that has given you financial stability. However, you realize some of the company's values are different from your own. How could this have been avoided? How can you rectify this situation going forward?

Activities

1. Log in to your university website and find the school's mission statement. Explain the mission statement. Does the campus mission statement embody your values and beliefs? Why or why not? What about your academic department's mission statement? Why or why not?

2. Interview one of your college professors. Ask them what their philosophy of education is. Explain what fundamental values or beliefs they mentioned. How does this compare to your philosophy?

3. Watch the TED Talk by Sam Berns. What is his philosophy of life? What health and wellness philosophy is he representing?

Weblinks

https://www.ted.com/talks/sam_berns_my_philosophy_for_a_happy_life

Sam Berns: My Philosophy for a Happy Life

Sam Berns, an American activist born with a rare genetic disorder called progeria, talks about how obstacles did not stop him from taking charge of his happiness.

https://www.nchec.org/responsibilities-and-competencies

NCHEC Responsibilities and Competencies for Health Education Specialists

The NCHEC websites help you navigate through all seven areas of responsibility and explain the daily tasks and characteristics of each.

References

American Cancer Society. (2017). *Mission statement.* Retrieved from https://www.cancer.org/about-us/who-we-are/mission-statements.html

Bensley, L. B. (1993). This I believe: A philosophy of health education. *The Eta Sigma Gamma Monograph Series, 11*(1), 1–7.

Berns, S. (2014). My philosophy for a happy life. [Video file]. Retrieved from https://www.ted.com/talks/sam_berns_my_philosophy_for_a_happy_life

Gambescia, S. F. (2007). 2007 SOPHE presidential address: Discovering a philosophy of health education. *Health Education and Behavior, 34*(5), 718–722.

Greenburg, J. S. (1978). Health education as freeing. *Health Education, 9*(2), 20–21.

National Commission for Health Education Credentialing, Inc. (2019). *Code of ethics.* Retrieved from https://www.nchec.org/code-of-ethics

Rash, J. K. (1985). Philosophical bases for health education. *Health Education, 16*(3), 48–49.

Schonfeld, Z. (2016). Remember that time Bill Clinton fired his surgeon general for encouraging masturbation education? Retrieved from https://www.newsweek.com/remember-time-bill-clinton-fired-his-surgeon-general-encouraging-masturbation-423302

Welle, H. M., Russell, R. D., & Kittleson, M. J. (1995). Philosophical trends in health education: Implications for the 21st century. *Journal of Health Education, 26* (6), 326–333.

Credits

Fig. 8.1: Source: https://commons.wikimedia.org/wiki/File:Joycelyn_Elders_official_photo_portrait.jpg.
Fig. 8.2: Source: http://canyonwalkerconnections.com/c-everett-koop-a-hero-during-the-aids-crisis/.
Fig. 8.3: Source: https://gracesalt.wordpress.com/2015/07/03/physical-emotional-social-spiritual-scale/.
Fig. 8.4: Source: https://twitter.com/sophetweets/status/1038064800042045447.
Fig. 8.5: Source: https://www.iaa.govt.nz/for-advisers/adviser-tools/ethics-toolkit/personal-beliefs-values-attitudes-and-behaviour/.

CHAPTER 9

Ethics and Professionalism in Health Education and Health Promotion

CHAPTER KEY

Authentic Learning: **using problem-solving of real-life scenarios to explore and discuss content and concepts.**

Collaboration: **working with content from other organizations or peers.**

Knowledge: **the theoretical or practical understanding of a concept.**

Practice: **applications of ideas or concepts.**

Reflection: **contemplation and meditation.**

Chapter Objectives

Upon completion of this chapter and participating in the critical thinking questions at the end, you should be able to master the following:

- **Define** ethics (*knowledge and reflection*).

- **Differentiate** between ethics and morality (*knowledge and reflection*).

- **Explain** ethical theories (*knowledge and reflection*).

- **Describe** the ethical areas of responsibility (*knowledge, reflection, practice, and collaboration*).

- **Outline** the steps in ethical decision-making (*authentic learning, reflection, practice, and collaboration*).

- **Explain** and **identify** how ethics is used in the health and wellness profession (*authentic learning, reflection, practice, and collaboration*).

Chapter Links to the Areas of Responsibility of a Health Educator/Health Promotion Professional

- Area of Responsibility IV: Evaluation and Research

- Area of Responsibility V: Advocacy

- Area of Responsibility VI: Communication

- Area of Responsibility VII: Leadership and Management

- Area of Responsibility VIII: Ethics and Professionalism

Introduction

Ethics impacts our lives every day. We continually see ethical issues play out on television and in social media, newspapers, magazines, etc. These ethical issues, such as abortion, the death penalty, genetic engineering, and reproductive issues, impact society, communities, and individuals drastically. As health educators, we have a responsibility to reach the highest possible standards of conduct and to encourage the ethical behavior of those with whom we work (NCHEC, 2020). This chapter will look at ethical perspectives and different approaches that can be used when making moral decisions. These tools will help health educators in identifying and clarifying problems and encourage them to view certain situations from multiple different vantage points. We will also look at the components of ethical decision-making, such as moral judgment, moral motivation, and honest character, and how these approaches will help in our ethical decision-making processes. Lastly, we will discuss the code of ethics of health education specialists and how we, as professionals, must act ethically in our own lives and careers.

The Terminology of Ethics

Ethics is known as the philosophical study of "right" and "wrong" or "good" and "bad" and is known as what humans ought to do or what our social system expects from us. **Morality** is our principles and the development of our own moral beliefs and moral conduct—the activity of making choices and deciding, judging, justifying, and defending those actions. Ethics is known as the study of morality (Morrison, 2006).

Often, we hear the word "ethics" interchangeably with terms such as "morals" and "morality" (see **Figure 9.1**), and that is because both ethics and morals have ancient Greek and

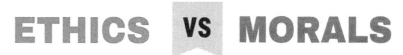

In most cases, when any one of us does something, we try to act according to what society believes is right. More often, we listen closely to what our own beliefs about right or wrong are telling us, even if they're different from society's views. These two have to do with ethics and morals.

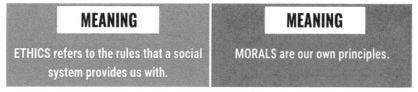

MEANING	MEANING
ETHICS refers to the rules that a social system provides us with.	MORALS are our own principles.

Figure 9.1 *The Difference Between Ethics and Morals.*

Latin roots in the words *ethos* and *mores*, and both mean *"character"* (White, 1988). One's character can be tested when faced with an **ethical issue** or **a moral dilemma**. Ethical issues and dilemmas force us to think systematically and encourage us to look at different viewpoints regarding an issue. These types of ethical dilemmas may pose as: Should a parent have the right to refuse immunizations for their child? Does public safety supersede an individual's rights (Lindsey-Henderson, 2016)? Should elder Americans be sacrificed amid the coronavirus pandemic?

Professional ethics is known as "actions that are right and wrong in the workplace and are of public matter. Professional moral principles are not statements of taste or preference; they tell practitioners what they ought to do and what they ought not to do" (Feeney & Freeman, 1999, p. 6). Ethical behavior is expected of professionals, and you will often find that many professions have their own sets of ethical standards that you are required to follow.

Health Educators' Ethical Areas of Responsibility

Health education specialists have their own **code of ethics** that provides each specialist with a set of ethical standards. Health education specialists are dedicated to excellence within the professional practice of promoting individual, family, organizational, and community health (NCHEC, 2020). The Health Education Code of Ethics provides a basis for shared professional values. The responsibility of all health education specialists is to reach the highest possible standards of conduct and to encourage the ethical behavior of all those with whom they work (NCHEC, 2020).

There are six critical ethical standards stated in the code of ethics for health educators:

> Article I: Responsibility to the Public
> Article II: Responsibility to the Profession
> Article III: Responsibility to Employers
> Article IV: Responsibility in the Delivery of Health Education
> Article V: Responsibility in Evaluation and Research
> Article VI: Responsibility in Professional Preparation (NCHEC, 2020).

It is important to note that our values and morals may guide us in our day-to-day activities, but they may not be sufficient to guide our professional behavior. The areas of responsibility noted above will help guide us in professional ethics. For example, as a health educator, you have an obligation to the public because our ultimate goal is to educate individuals for the sole purpose of promoting, maintaining, and improving quality of life for individuals, families, and communities (NCHEC, 2020). You may be faced with conflict when issues arise amongst different groups, individuals, agencies, and organizations. Still, as a health educator, you must consider all issues and their consequences and give priority to those that promote wellness and quality of life (NCHEC, 2020). In addition to our responsibility toward the public, we have a responsibility toward our profession of health education, health promotion, and wellness. We are responsible for our professional behavior as well as the reputation of our profession, which means that we must promote ethical behavior and conduct amongst our colleagues and peers. This responsibility to the profession is also linked to our responsibility to our employers. As health educators, we must recognize the boundaries of our professional competence and account for our professionalism, activities, and actions while in the workplace (NCHEC, 2020).

Health educators also have a responsibility to provide the most up-to-date health information. In doing this, our delivery of health education must respect the rights, dignity, and confidentiality of all people. This means we must adopt strategies and methods to meet the needs of diverse populations and communities (NCHEC, 2020). To meet these needs, we have a responsibility to contribute to the health field through research and evaluation. When planning and conducting research or evaluation, health educators do so following federal and state laws and regulations, organizational and institutional policies, and professional standards (NCHEC, 2020). It is important to remember that evaluation and research should never cause mental, physical, or emotional harm, nor should they delay products or services that could improve one's health and wellness. To ensure our research is in agreeance with federal and state laws and regulations, researchers should have research ethics and compliance training.

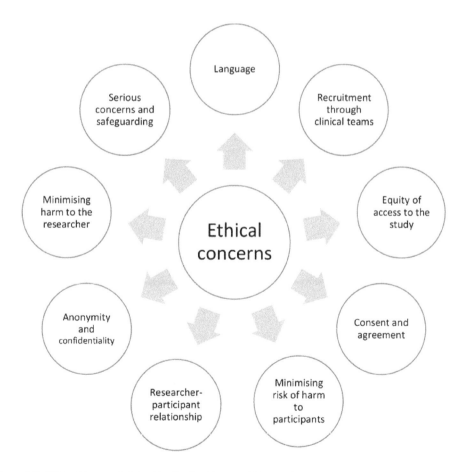

Figure 9.2 *Ethical Issues Related to Evaluation and Research*
Adapted from Mitchell, Slowther, Coad, & Dale, 2018.

Lastly, health educators have a responsibility in professional preparation, meaning that those involved in the preparation and training of health educators must accord learners the same respect and treatment given other groups by providing quality education that benefits the profession and the public (NCHEC, 2020).

How Does Ethics Affect Our Health?

Acting ethically can bring purpose to one's life and can provide a better society for all. McGrath (1994) found that those who act ethically tend to live healthier and emotionally satisfying lives. Additionally, human flourishing requires resources and the appropriate social conditions necessary to secure equal opportunities for all (APHA, 2020). Acting ethically can improve health for individuals and communities and can aid in achieving equity in health status for our nation.

Health equity means everyone can reach their optimal level of health, that everyone has access to resources and services that optimize conditions in which we are born, grow, live, learn, work, and age (APHA, 2020; see **Figure 9.3**). When you think about ethics and the health challenges that many worldwide are faced with, it raises questions about health resource allocation, health technologies, decision-making in clinical care, and public health. Does everyone have the same access to healthcare, services, education, products, and finances?

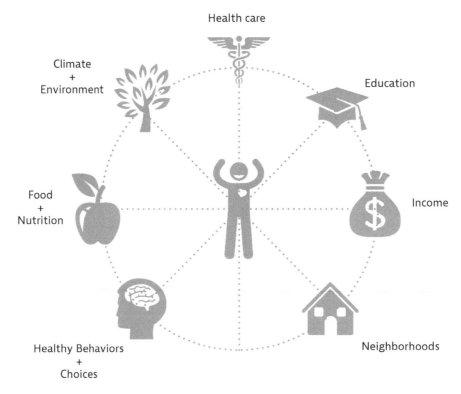

Figure 9.3 *American Public Health Association's Advancement of Public Health Ethics in Practice.*

Ethical Principles

To understand the ethical theory, you must understand the common set of ethical principles that decision makers use to make a successful decision. The four ethical principles consist of respect for autonomy, beneficence, nonmaleficence, and justice (See **Figure 9.4**).

Principles of Ethics

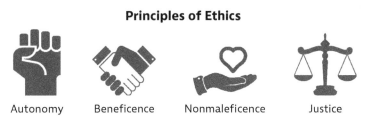

Autonomy   Beneficence   Nonmaleficence   Justice

Figure 9.4 *The Four Ethical Principles.*

The principle of **autonomy** states that decision-making should focus on allowing individuals to make their own decisions based on their own lives (Coggon & Miola, 2011). This means people should have control over their own lives because they are the only ones who understand their chosen type of lifestyle. This is also known as the principle of human dignity (Greenberg, 2001). **Beneficence** helps guides the decision maker to do what is "right" and what is considered "good." This principle strives to achieve "good" because we all benefit from good (Chonko, 2015). **Nonmaleficence** means the least harm and deals with situations where no choice seems to be the most beneficial. Decision makers will choose to do the least harm as possible and harm a few people (Page, 2012). The last ethical principle looks at **justice**, where decision makers should focus on actions that are fair to all involved. This means the ethical decisions we make should be consistent and justified within the scenario (Velasquez, Andre, Shanks, & Meyer, 2020).

Ethical Theories

Ethical theories help provide a foundation for our decision-making by helping guide us in seeing different vantage points. Each theory has a different decision-making style with different rules. This is because not everyone makes the same decisions in the same way. We use ethical theory to guide us in making a decision when in an ethical dilemma. Using an ethical theory can lead to the most ethically correct resolution. There are four ethical theories, known as utilitarianism, deontology, rights, and virtues (Chonko, 2015).

Utilitarianism determines right from wrong by focusing on outcomes and is based on the premise that ethical choices should be based on their consequences. People generally think about the likely outcomes of their decisions when determining what to do. Utilitarianism holds that the most ethical choice is the one that will produce the greatest good for the greatest number: the end does justify the means (Posner, 1979). For example, it is okay to tell a lie to save a friend from a murderer.

Deontology states that consequences do not matter. This means that someone will follow the rules and obligations of society because it is what is considered ethically correct. For example, a deontologist would not tell a lie to save a friend from murder because telling a lie is considered "wrong" in society's eyes (Pozgar, 2013). Someone who adheres to this theory is very consistent and will make decisions based on their set of duties.

Rights, as an ethical theory, is based on the rights established by society. Rights are considered to be ethically correct, "right," or "good" because they are endorsed by society and the population. This theory also bestows rights upon others (Kiran, 2007). For example, you checked out a book from the school library to do your research paper. You now have the right to that book for the time you checked out the book. This theory does have its conflicts because it is the society that determines what rights it wants to uphold and give to its citizens. For example, in America, people have the right to choose their religion because this right is upheld in the Constitution.

The **virtue** ethical theory judges individuals by their character rather than by actions that may deviate from the individual's normal behavior (Chonko, 2015). For example, a student plagiarized a paper and the teacher detected it; the teacher who knows the student well and understands their character will judge them accordingly. If the student is one who normally follows the rules, is in good academic standing, and has never plagiarized before, the teacher would be more lenient with the student. Conversely, a person who has a reputation for academic misconduct is more likely to be judged harshly for plagiarizing because of their past behavior (Chonko, 2015).

	Utilitarian Ethics	Deontological Ethics	Virtue Ethics
definition	the greatest good for the greatest number of people	the idea that people should be treated with dignity and respect	considering what virtues make a good public relations professionals
application	making a decision based on what will benefit the majority	identifying one's duty and acting accordingly	making a decision in light of those favored virtues
pros & cons	Con: decision-makers are forced to guess the outcome of their choice Con: harming a minority and benefitting a majority doesn't build mutually beneficial relationships Con: it is not always possible to predict the outcome of a decision	Con: there may be disagreement about the principles involved in the decision Con: the possibility of making a "right" choice with bad consequence Con: the possibility of a conflict in duties Pros: strongest model for applied public relations ethics	Con: misses the importance obligations to client and publics Con: the possibility of a conflict in virtues

Figure 9.5 *Pros and Cons of Ethical Theory.*

How to Make Ethical Decisions

As health educators, we must possess the appropriate requisite knowledge and skills to make ethical decisions. In addition to using the ethical principles and the ethical theories, several steps aid in providing a framework for making ethical decisions. It is important to remember that the ethical decision-making process should begin long before any ethical dilemmas arise. Below is the seven-step ethical decision-making process (adapted from Davis, 1999, pp. 166–167).

1. **State the Problem**

   a. What is the problem or ethical issue you are tackling? Is there something about this decision that makes me uneasy? Do I have a conflict of interest?

2. **Check the Facts**

   a. After stating the problem, look closer. Is it a problem that could be easily solved upon closer examination? Or is it possible that this could evolve into a bigger issue?

   b. Think about those who are involved. Could this ethical issue involve laws, policies, professional codes, or other constraints?

3. **Identify Relevant Factors**

   a. Internal: are there any factors intrapersonally that you would need to account for?

   b. External: are there any factors interpersonally that you would need to account for?

4. **Develop a List of Options**

   a. Weigh your options.

   b. Be imaginative. What theory could best help with this issue?

   c. Who could you bring in to help you with this issue? Who could you go to?

5. **Test the Options** (Use some of the following tests)

   a. *Harm test*: Does this option do less harm than the alternatives?

   b. *Publicity test*: Would I want my choice of this option published in the newspaper?

   c. *Defensibility test*: Could I defend my choice of this option before a congressional committee or committee of peers?

   d. *Reversibility test*: Would I still think this option was a good choice if I were adversely affected by it?

   e. *Colleague test*: What do my colleagues say when I describe my problem and suggest this option as my solution?

   f. *Professional test*: What might my profession's governing body for ethics say about this option?

   g. *Organization test*: What does my company's ethics officer or legal counsel say about this?

6. Make a Choice

a. Consider steps 1–5. What were the outcomes? What is the best decision?

7. Review Steps 1–6

a. Evaluate how you came to your conclusions.
b. Could you have more support next time?
c. Are there any cautions you would take next time?
d. Having made a decision based on the process above, how are you now prepared to *act* on this decision?

(adapted from Davis, 1999, pp. 166–167).

Ethical Issues in Health Education and Health Promotion

As mentioned before, ethical considerations take place in every aspect of our lives, so it is obvious that health education and health promotion would be no different. Some of the ethical issues we face in health education and health promotion are part of the profession, such as ethical issues with clients, using interventions, protecting patients' rights, etc.

Privacy protections provide valuable benefits to society. Privacy is used in health research and is vital in improving human health and healthcare (Institute of Medicine, 2009). Additionally, protecting patients' privacy and their rights is essential in ethical research. Privacy is very important because of personal autonomy, individuality, respect, and dignity and worth as human beings. Can you remember a time when your privacy was not protected? How did that make you feel?

The Health Insurance Portability and Accountability Act (HIPPA) helps reduce healthcare fraud and abuse and mandates standards for healthcare information in electronic billing and other processes. Furthermore, it requires the protection and confidential handling of protected health information (DHCS, 2020).

The Genetic Information Nondiscrimination Act (GINA) prohibits genetic discrimination in health insurance and employment. However, GINA does not prevent discrimination in forms of insurance related to life, disability, or long-term care (NIH, 2020).

Summary

From this chapter, we can see that ethics affects all aspects of our daily lives. We are constantly being faced with ethical dilemmas and issues, both in our personal and professional lives. Specifically, as health educators, we must have a basic understanding of ethics, ethical theories, and principles to aid in our decision-making processes when faced with certain scenarios in our field of work. The steps in ethical decision-making can help health educators look at all vantage points and determine what is "right" and "wrong." This chapter investigates health equity and how ethics is also an important part of reaching an optimal level of health. Overall, acting ethically can bring purpose to our lives and provide a better society for all.

Review Questions

1. Explain the differences between ethics and morals.

2. What are the key ethical principles discussed in this chapter? What does each of the principles mean?

3. What is the difference between utilitarianism and deontology? What types of ethical dilemmas would be most appropriate to use these theories?

4. What does the term "professional ethics" mean? How does the term "professional ethics" connect to our code of ethics as health educators?

Case Scenario

You recently graduated and are using your free time to volunteer at a local hospital. You go room to room with the smiles cart brightening patients' days and providing emotional support. While in the elevator, you are accompanied by three nurses and two other hospital visitors. You hear the nurses talking about a patient named Susie Kemp, a patient on the third floor. They are talking about her condition and other protected information. As a recent graduate, you think back to your course on professional ethics and our code of ethics as health educators. Based on this chapter, what did the nurses violate? What responsibility areas from the code of ethics did the nurses violate? Who should you contact about this situation? Should a supervisor be notified?

Critical Thinking Questions

1. Ethical dilemmas are never easy. How would you deal with a coworker acting unethically in the workplace? Would it change your opinion if this was not your coworker's normal behavior? What type of ethical theory does this represent?

2. Think of a time when you were faced with an ethical dilemma. How would you address that dilemma now using the seven steps of ethical decision-making?

3. After reading through the code of ethics, is anything missing? Would you add anything to The Health Education Specialist Code of Ethics? Would you remove anything?

4. Which ethical theory do you most identify with? Do you approach most ethical dilemmas and issues through this lens? Why or why not?

Activities

1. You are on a sinking ship, and there is only one lifeboat available. The maximum occupancy is 8 persons and will sink if overoccupied. Waiting to board the lifeboat are nine adults and one child. You must decide who stays and who boards the boat. Be prepared to defend your decision. Occupants:

    a. You are one of the occupants
    b. A young mother and her infant son
    c. 75-year-old retired physician
    d. The wife of the retired physician
    e. Pregnant female (this counts as one person)
    f. A male professional athlete
    g. A priest
    h. A lifeguard
    i. The captain of the ship

Who did you decide to keep off the boat? Why did you make this decision? Do you feel like your decision was ethical? Was there any bias in how you responded?

2. You see your friend cheating on their certified health education specialist exam (CHES exam). Using the virtue ethical theory, how would you go about dealing with this dilemma? Would you tell the instructor? Why or why not?

3. To research in the health field, you must have training on how to deal with human subjects. Log on to https://about.citiprogram.org/en/homepage/ and register with your local institution. Once you have logged in, explore one of the research areas, such as social and behavioral science. These foundational pieces of training in human subject research include the historical development of human subject protections, ethical issues, and current regulatory information regarding research.

Web Links

https://about.citiprogram.org/en/homepage/

CITI Training

This site provides several pieces of training on research ethics and compliance training for dealing with human subjects.

https://www.nchec.org/code-of-ethics

NCHEC Code of Ethics

The code of ethics for a health education specialist details each responsibility area that allows specialists to encourage ethical behavior for individuals and communities.

https://www.apha.org/-/media/files/pdf/membergroups/ethics/code_of_ethics.ashx

APHA Public Health Code of Ethics

This document details the Public Health Code of Ethics, which is a professional set of standards that relay the expectations intended for public health practitioners in the field.

https://www.hhs.gov/hipaa/index.html

U.S. Department of Health and Human Services

This website details health information privacy, including an overview of HIPPA.

https://www.ethics.org/

Ethics & Compliance Initiative (ECI)

The Ethics & Compliance Initiative (ECI) is a nonprofit organization that empowers its members across the globe to operate their businesses at the highest levels of integrity.

http://cnheo.org/ethics.html

Coalition of National Health Education Organizations (CNHEO)

The Coalition outlines the code of ethics and provides various documents that show changes made over the years.

References

American Public Health Association. (2020a). *Health equity*. Retrieved from https://www.apha.org/topics-and-issues/health-equity

American Public Health Association (2020). *Ethics*. Retrieved from https://www.apha.org/apha-communities/member-sections/ethics

Chonko, L. (2015). *Ethical theories*. Austin: University of Texas.

Coggon, J., & Miola, J. (2011). Autonomy, liberty, and medical decision-making. *The Cambridge Law Journal*, *70*(3), 523–547. doi: 10.1017/s0008197311000845

Davis, M. (1999). *Ethics and the university*. New York: Routledge.

DHCS. (2019). *What is HIPPA?* Retrieved from https://www.dhcs.ca.gov/formsandpubs/laws/hipaa/Pages/1.00WhatisHIPAA.aspx

Greenberg, J. S. (2001). *The code of ethics for the health education profession: A case study book*. Boston, MA: Jones & Bartlett Publishers.

Institute of Medicine of the National Academics. (2009). *Beyond the HIPAA privacy rule: Enhancing privacy, improving health through research*. Nass, S. J., Levit, L. A., Gostin, L. O. (Eds.). Washington, DC: National Academies Press.

Kiran, D. R. (2007). *Professional ethics and human values*. New Delhi: Tate McGraw-Hill.

Lindsey-Henderson, S. (2016, September). Ethics in hearing healthcare: Strategies in ethical solutions. *Shaping the Future 65th Annual IHS Convention & Expo*, Chicago, IL. Retrieved from https://ihsinfo.org/IhsV2/Convention2016/pdf/seminar/09%20Ethics%20in%20Hearing%20Healthcare.pdf

McGrath, E. Z. (1994). *The art of ethics: A psychology of ethical beliefs*. Chicago, IL: Loyola University Press.

Mitchell, S., Slowther, A.-M., Coad, J., & Dale, J. (2018). The journey through care: Study protocol for a longitudinal qualitative interview study to investigate the healthcare experiences and preferences of children and young people with life-limiting and life-threatening conditions and their families in the West Midlands, UK. *BMJ Open, 8*(1). doi: 10.1136/bmjopen-2017-018266

Morrison, E. E. (2006). *Ethics in health administration: A practical approach for decision makers*. Sudbury, MA: Jones & Bartlett.

National Institutes of Health: Genetics Home Reference. (2020). *What is genetic discrimination*? Retrieved from https://ghr.nlm.nih.gov/primer/testing/discrimination

National Commission for Health Education Credentialing, Inc. (2020). *Health education code of ethics*. Retrieved from https://www.nchec.org/code-of-ethics

Page, K. (2012). The four principles: Can they be measured and do they predict ethical decision making? *BMC Medical Ethics, 13*(1). doi: 10.1186/1472-6939-13-10

Posner, R. (1979). Utilitarianism, economics, and legal theory. *Journal of Legal Studies, 8,* 103–40.

Pozgar, J. H. (2013). *Legal and ethical issues for health professionals* (3rd ed.). Burlington, MA: Jones and Bartlett Learning.

Velasquez, M., Andre, C., Shanks, T., & Meyer, M. (2020). Justice and Fairness. Retrieved from https://www.scu.edu/ethics/ethics-resources/ethical-decision-making/justice-and-fairness/

White, T. I. (1988). Right and wrong: A brief guide to understanding ethics. Englewood Cliffs, NJ: Prentice-Hall.

Credits

CHAPTER 10

The Health Education Specialist

CHAPTER KEY

Authentic Learning: **using problem-solving of real-life scenarios to explore and discuss content and concepts.**

Knowledge: **the theoretical or practical understanding of a concept.**

Reflection: **contemplation or meditation.**

Practice: **applications of ideas or concepts.**

Leadership: **the act of leading a group or organization.**

Collaboration: **working with content from other organizations or peers.**

Social Justice: **fair and just relations between individuals and society.**

Chapter Objectives

Upon completion of this chapter and participating in the critical thinking questions at the end, you should be able to:

- **List** and **describe** the eight areas of responsibility for health educators (*knowledge, reflection, practice, and collaboration*).

- **Explain** and **discuss** the history behind health educators (*knowledge, reflection, practice, and collaboration*).

- **Define** and **explain** what CHES is and what it stands for (*knowledge, reflection, practice, and collaboration*).

Chapter Links to the Areas of Responsibility of a Health Educator/Health Promotion Professional

- Area of Responsibility I: Assessment of Needs Capacity
- Area of Responsibility II: Planning
- Area of Responsibility III: Implementation
- Area of Responsibility IV: Evaluation and Research
- Area of Responsibility V: Advocacy
- Area of Responsibility VI: Communication
- Area of Responsibility VII: Leadership and Management
- Area of Responsibility VIII: Ethics and Professionalism

Introduction

As we learned in Chapter 3, health education and wellness has been around since the earliest humans, yet certification in health education did not get its start until 1978. The health education profession has been validating competencies that are used for professional credentials, preparation, and development for years. The current roles and responsibilities of a health educator are outlined in this chapter, starting with the historical background of how health education and wellness got its start in the United States and then identifying credentialing bodies, the certification for health education specialists, and the current roles and responsibilities that make up a health educator in today's workforce. These responsibilities and competencies provide a full description of our profession, illustrating the skills necessary to perform the daily tasks of a health education specialist (NCHEC, 2020). In the following pages, you will learn about the eight areas of responsibility for health education specialists, which include competencies such as planning, evaluation, administration, communication, and promotion.

Who Are Health Educators?

Have you ever been asked "What is health promotion? What is health education? What is it exactly that you do?" or "What kind of job can you get after your degree?" If you have been asked any of these questions, like many other health educators, you will be able to outline precisely what it is we do after reading this chapter.

Certified Health Education Specialist or Health Educator

A **health educator** is a professionally prepared individual who possesses knowledge and skills based upon theories and research to promote behavior change within individuals and communities (Bruening et al., 2018). Health educators provide information on wellness and health-related issues in a variety of different settings. They can assess health training needs, plan health education programs, implement health education programs, and evaluate health education programs. Some may specialize in a given health area or illness, while others may work in a specific system. For instance, you may find health educators working at the government level for county health departments, local community organizations, businesses, hospitals, schools, and other governmental agencies. They often do the following tasks:

- Perform health training and needs assessments

- Design and develop health education programs

- Publish health education materials, information papers, and grant proposals

- Develop health education curricula

- Teach health in public or private schools (Bruening et al., 2018).

Health educators are uniquely positioned to address public health needs and issues by using their training and competencies in the application of behavioral theories across a wide range of interventions designed to improve population health (Bruening et al., 2018). Often, we see health educators using a holistic philosophy approach (discussed in Chapter 8) to aid in changing health behaviors, implementing evidence-based interventions, and adapting to the ever-changing population (Bruening et al., 2018).

How to Become a Certified Health Education Specialist

To become a certified health education specialist, one needs to obtain the required certification credentials. A **certification** "is a process by which a professional organization grants recognition to an individual who, upon completion of a competency-based curriculum, can demonstrate a predetermined standard of performance" (Cleary, 1995, p. 39). Certification is available for all health educators who have met the required academic preparation qualifications and successfully passed competency-based examinations administered by the National Commission for Health Education Credentialing, Inc. (NCHEC; NCHEC, 2020). The **Certified Health Education Specialist (CHES)** examination (CHES®) consists of 165 multiple-choice questions that are focused on the eight areas of responsibility for health education specialists. Once certified, you are then recognized with CHES credentials, which can be added after your name and academic degree. The Master Certified Health Education Specialist (MCHES) credentials are for those interested in obtaining an advanced certification. The MCHES exam (MCHES®) also focuses on the eight areas of responsibility but is designed for experienced specialists with at least 5 years of experience (NCHEC, 2018). The CHES exam has met national standards in credentialing and has been accredited by the National Commission of Certifying Agencies since 2008 (NCHEC, 2018).

Areas of Responsibility of a Health Educator

There were seven areas of responsibility that were initially discussed by the National Task Force on the Preparation and Practice of Health Education (1985). Since then, they have been revised with the addition of certification (1989), a code of ethics (2000), competency updates (2005 and 2015) and several revisions to the materials (2005, 2006, 2007, 2008, 2010, 2011, and 2015; NCHEC, 2018).

The responsibilities were verified by the 2015 Health Education Specialist Practice Analysis (HESPA) project and serve as the basis of both the CHES® and the MCHES® exams (NCHEC, 2018). This led to the terminology change of "health education" to "health education/health promotion." Each of these responsibilities has competencies and sub-competencies, which together describe the role of Health Education Specialists and their duties in the field (NCHEC, 2018). As of 2020, the seven areas of responsibility were updated to **eight** containing a comprehensive set of **competencies**, and sub-competencies defined the role of the health education specialist (NCHEC, 2020). These Responsibilities were verified by the 2020 Health Education Specialist Practice Analysis II (HESPA II 2020) project and serve as the basis of the CHES® and MCHES® exam beginning 2021 (NCHEC, 2020).

The most current version describing the Health Education Specialist's responsibilities, competencies, and sub-competencies are stated in the Health Education Job Analysis (Areas of Responsibilities, Competencies, and Sub-competencies for Health Education Specialists, 2015) (Table 10.1).

Table 10.1 THE EIGHT AREAS OF RESPONSIBILITY

Area I	Assessment of Needs and Capacity
Area II	Planning
Area III	Implementation
Area IV	Evaluation and Research
Area V	Advocacy
Area VI	Communication
Area VII	Leadership and Management
Area VIII	Ethics and Professionalism

Responsibility I: Assessment of Needs and Capacity

In health education/health promotion, it is essential for the Health Promotion Specialist to know their target population. This includes the demographics, size, current assets, culture, needs, and desires of the target population. Once there is an understanding of the target population, and the Health Promotion Specialist can differentiate between what the target population has, or assets and capacity. What they need or desire, it is easier to develop health goals (McKenzie, Neiger, & Thackeray, 2017). As described in chapter 7, when done well, this is a very involved process that requires commitment, immersion, and open-mindedness, and is termed **needs assessment** of the target population. A needs assessment can be defined as "the process of identifying, analyzing, and prioritizing the needs of a priority population" (McKenzie, Neiger, & Thackeray, 2017, p. 68).

When discussing a needs assessment, it is imperative to determine if the needs are individual or community-wide. Identifying the level of interaction first, individual or community will help the Health Promotion Specialist plan health services that meet the greater need of the target population (Wright, Williams, & Wilkinson, 1998). If the needs of the community are ignored, the majority of the target population will not benefit from the health services. For example, if a smoking cessation program is being implemented in a community where only 10% of the members smoke, but there is a high rate of risky sexual behavior (85%). The Health Promotion Specialist should change its focus to impact the greater good or majority.

The needs assessment process involves collecting primary and secondary data. **Primary data** is collected directly from the source. In the case of a needs assessment of a target population, the Health Promotion Specialist can go directly to an individual of that population. To collect this data, the Health Promotion Specialist could administer a survey, conduct an interview, or hold a focus group to get the most accurate information regarding the individuals within the target population.

Secondary data is information that already exists. Another Health Promotion Specialist, doctor, researcher, etc. may have previously collected information regarding the target population, using the same methods previously mentioned, and analyzed the data. Other preexisting data can be from the census, which identifies information such as household income and size, race, ethnicity, gender, employment rates, etc. This data is useful because it can provide you with a starting point in terms of gaining background information, in addition to lending itself to help identify patterns and trends that are present within the community.

So, which type of data is better? Both primary and secondary data have their advantages and disadvantages. Secondary data is already available, and you do not need to spend much time or money to access it. However, it may not directly answer the questions of the Health Promotion Specialist. Primary data will explain the specific questions the Health Promotion Specialist has, but it will take time to collect and analyze (McKenzie, Neiger, & Thackeray, 2017).

Some techniques for collecting data are:

- **Interviews:** Interviews are the most intimate interactions that occur between two parties during data collection. The interaction occurs between the interviewer and the interviewee, in which a series of questions are posed and answered. There is some discrepancy about whether or not the interviewers enter the meeting with questions already prepared to ask the community members. Taylor, Bogdan, and DeVault (2015) claim, "Until we enter the field, we do not know what questions to ask or how to ask them" (p. 30). Generally, it is recommended that you prepare a set of questions to work from and use your best judgment on how to move forward when conducting the interview. However, this is dependent on the type of interview you are conducting; formal or informal. Structured interviews have a specific script you must follow, while informal interviews allow for more of a conversation between the interviewer and interviewee.

  Regardless of which approach you choose is best for your initiative and target population, it is essential to be knowledgeable of the community so that your questions are based on grounded information, and also that you are open to strategically veering from intended questions when necessary. When crafting these questions, you want them to be open-ended. Any question that elicits a "yes" or "no" response does not successfully provide you with the details needed for an explanation. With that being said, if you do find your interviewee responding in the "yes" or "no" fashion, be prepared to ask follow-up questions in order to access as much information as possible.

- **Focus Groups:** Focus groups differ from interviews because they tend to involve a greater number of people. Krueger and Casey (2015), describe focus groups as generally being comprised of five to eight people but can vary in size from four to twelve participants. This qualitative practice is less about one person taking the role of an interviewer, and more about facilitating discussion amongst the group members. It is imperative that the facilitator prepares questions and prompts that have a focused purpose. Questions of an open-ended nature should begin the discussion to get participants comfortable and geared towards the topic at hand. As questions progress, they should become "more specific–more focused" in order to gain insight and data about specific areas (Krueger and Casey, 2015). When hosting a meeting that involves a large number of people, it is important that the facilitator(s) find a balance between allowing participants to respond freely, but also refocusing conversations back to the intended purpose, so that you are able to gain meaningful information.

- **Surveys:** Surveys, according to Fowler (2014), are "fundamentally a matter of asking a sample of people from a population a set of questions and using the answers to describe that population" (p. ix). Surveys can aid in health promotion initiatives in different ways. Surveys can be administered towards the beginning of the process as a means to collect quantitative data in order to gain background information about your target population, which can help aid you in the needs assessment. You can also use surveys to collect more in-depth responses. If you are looking for more qualitative data, you want to be careful to avoid solely "yes"/"no" questions, because you will only be generating more quantitative data. You should work to create open-ended questions, and even format surveys with a response area that is blank or has lines, rather than offering multiple-choice or checklist style framing. When respondents see lines or blank boxes, they are more likely to provide details in their responses that you may not have even anticipated as being a likely answer. While creating and administering surveys takes careful planning, they do offer your target population flexibility. For example, some individuals may be unable or unwilling to appear in person at designated times for an interview or focus group. Furthermore, there may be some people that do not feel comfortable (despite the specialist's best efforts) sharing ideas and concerns, and wish to retain their anonymity, which surveys have the ability to offer. Lastly, due to the fact that surveys can be distributed in person via a paper copy or electronically via online platforms, be sure to account for accessibility to the survey amongst the target group.

- **Observation:** There are three main approaches to observation: complete, participant, and researcher. In complete observation, specialists take more of a back seat and are not actively involved in occurring situations. This practice tends to yield quantitative results because the observer is noting their surroundings without really being able to gain an understanding of why and how things are happening. Even though all three types of observation allow specialists to view the target population in their "natural context," participant and researcher observation can generate insights that other forms of research cannot" (Guest, Namey, Mitchell, 2013, p. 11). Participant and researcher observation allows the specialist to engage with members of the target population and typically happens over an extended period of time. As a participant and research observer, you are essentially acting as a member of that group as you collect pertinent data. The difference is, is that as a researcher observer, you disclose yourself as a researcher, while in participant observation, you do not disclose yourself as a researcher. In both approaches to observation, it is important to note things such as physical space, individuals present, dialogue, activities, body language, as well as any other practices and objects that are or are not present that may affect your initiative. While you would want to get permission to attend the non-public activities, some that you may consider observing are staff meetings, town hall sessions, organized community events, ceremonies, religious gatherings, conferences, etc.

Responsibility II: Planning

Once the Health Education Specialist has collected and analyzed the data, they should have a thorough understanding of the needs of their target population. The next step is to take that newly acquired information and begin the planning process for the health service/program. The steps in the planning process should always include (1) recruit stakeholders in the community, (2) establish goals and objectives for the health service, and (3) select a program design and create a plan to deliver it (Areas of Responsibilities, Competencies, and Sub-competencies for Health Education Specialists, 2015).

Before planning the actual health service/program, it is imperative first to recruit stakeholders within the community and allow them to be part of the planning and evaluating of the health service (Gilliam et al., 2002). Collaboration and open communication between the Health Promotion Specialist, her planning team, and leaders and members of the community will help establish a solid foundation and give the program a better chance of being effective at meeting the needs of the target population (Gilliam et al., 2002). You can further explore this process and significance in chapter 7.

Goals and objectives provide a set of standards of which the program is designed to meet. Although we often see the words used interchangeably, they are not synonymous. The term **goal** was defined by the Centers for Disease Control and Prevention as "A broad statement about the long-term expectation of what should happen as a result of your program (the desired outcome)" (Salabarría-Peña, Y., Apt, B., Walsh, 2007, p. 2) The goals are used as a foundation for developing the **objectives**, which are "statements describing the results to be achieved, and the manner in which they will be achieved." Generally, there are several objectives to address a single goal (Salabarría-Peña, Y., Apt, B., Walsh, 2007, p. 2). Creating goals and objectives with the stakeholders is ideal in laying out the plan of the health service/program.

As part of the planning process, the Health Education Specialist must identify the resources that they need and that are available in the target community. Some resources that should be considered are personnel, instructional resources, space, equipment, supplies, and financial resources (McKenzie, Neiger, & Thackeray, 2017). Personnel includes the individuals needed to carry out the program. This could be volunteers, support staff, or anyone associated with the program. Instructional resources would be material needed to teach the content of the health service. This could be a curriculum or any education material that is bought or created by the program planners. How much space is needed to carry out the program? And where will it be held? Equipment (computers, tools, hardware, tables, etc.) and supplies (office supplies) are a financial concern and should be considered in the planning process. All of the above may have a financial component to them and need to be factored into the budget and discussed when considering how the program is going to be funded.

Responsibility III: Implementation

After all of the planning, the implementation process is the time that is most exciting to Health Education Specialists. They are finally given the opportunity to offer the health program, or service, to the target population. However, it is essential that all of those on the implementation team follow that exact same protocol, so the program is implemented properly and without bias. Standardization of the implementation process will help reduce Type III Errors, or "failure to implement the health education intervention properly" (Basch et al., 1985).

As mentioned in Responsibility I, it is best practice to make sure the program is meeting the needs of the majority of the target population. However, we should also be taking into consideration the needs of the individuals of the population as well. To make sure the program is meeting the needs of the greatest number of individuals in the target population, the CDC (2015) suggests focusing the program implementation in the following four categories:

- Health-related Programs—opportunities available to employees at the workplace or through outside organizations to begin, change or maintain health behaviors.

- Health-related Policies—are formal or informal written statements that are designed to protect or promote employee health. Supportive workplace health policies affect large groups of workers simultaneously and make adopting healthy behaviors much easier. They can also create and foster a company culture of health.

- Health Benefits—part of an overall compensation package including health insurance coverage and other services or discounts regarding health (McLeroy et al., 1988).

- Environmental Support—refers to the physical factors at and near the workplace that help protect and enhance employee health.

Finally, as the program is up and running, it must be monitored to make sure everything is going as planned. At this time, evaluation should be conducted (Responsibility IV).

Responsibility IV: Evaluation and Research

Once the program is in place, evaluation of the health service should take place. There are two types of evaluation formative and summative evaluation. To ensure the program is running, a formal monitoring strategy, or **formative evaluation**, is designed during the planning process and executed during the implementation process of the program. Formative evaluation acts as quality control to ensure the program is progressing as planned (McKenzie, Neiger, & Thackeray, 2017). If the program is not following the set plan, the formative evaluation will help to identify small changes that should be made better to reach the goals and objectives of the program. Ultimately, this will help save money and time because the Health Promotion Specialist will not get to the end of the program and realize it wasn't successful.

As formative evaluation takes place as the program progresses, summative evaluation is conducted at the end of the program to determine program effectiveness. **Summative evaluation** is "any combination of measurements and judgments that permit conclusions to be drawn about impact, outcome, or benefits of a program method" (Green & Lewis, 1986, p. 336). Ultimately, summative evaluation is used to assess if the goals and objectives of the program have been met.

Formative and summative evaluation tools can range from focus groups, and personal interviews, to surveys and direct observation. As a Health Education Specialist, it is important to be aware of, and familiar with, all of the available evaluation tools, and to be able to determine the tools that will best measure the outcomes you expect from your health program. Without the proper evaluation method, the Health Education Specialist would not be able to determine if the program was effective and, therefore, would not have any information to disseminate to the stakeholders. Ultimately, conducting program evaluations will involve the stakeholders and increase the likelihood that they will continue to support the efforts of the program (MMWR, 1999).

The planning of the evaluation processes should occur during the overall program planning process (**Figure 10.1**). Once the evaluation design and tools are created, they are used to gather evidence on the program that determines the quality, efficiency, and effectiveness of the program (MMWR, 1999).

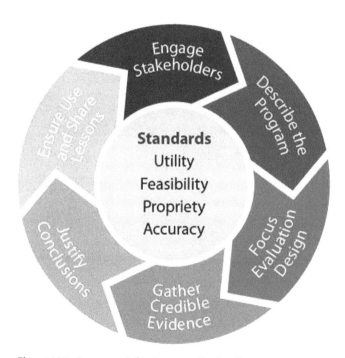

Figure 10.1 *Framework for Program Evaluation.*

The data that is collected during the evaluation process can be qualitative or quantitative. **Qualitative data** is "information presented in the narrative form used in the evaluation to provide detailed summaries of descriptions of observations, interactions, or verbal accounts (e.g., data from focus groups, in-depth interviews)" (McKenzie, Neiger, & Thackeray, 2017, p. 429). **Quantitative data** is "information expressed in numerical terms that can be compared on scales" (McKenzie, Neiger, & Thackeray, 2017, p. 429). A more detailed discussion of qualitative and quantitative data analysis can be viewed in chapter 7.

Once the data is collected, it must be analyzed, interpreted, and then implemented. Reports of the findings are created as a formal document to display and disseminate the information to the stakeholders and other appropriate parties (Cottrell, Girvan & McKenzie, 2008).

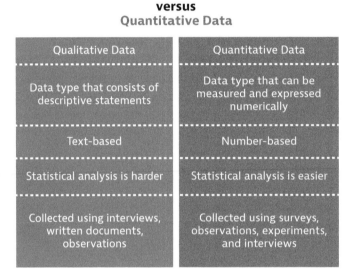

Qualitative Data
versus
Quantitative Data

Qualitative Data	Quantitative Data
Data type that consists of descriptive statements	Data type that can be measured and expressed numerically
Text-based	Number-based
Statistical analysis is harder	Statistical analysis is easier
Collected using interviews, written documents, observations	Collected using surveys, observations, experiments, and interviews

Figure 10.2 *Qualitative Data Vs. Quantitative Data Procedures.*

Responsibility V: Administer and Manage Health Education/Promotion

In this area of responsibility, a health educator must exercise organizational leadership by being able to conduct strategic planning within an organization, analyze the organization's culture in relation to health promotion program goals, and promote cooperation and feedback among personnel related to the program. In order for a health promotion program to be successful, the health educator must be able to consult stakeholders in administration and management. Health education specialists must be able to gain support from their stakeholders by explaining how the program goals align with the organizational structure, such as the mission, goals, and objectives. After gaining stakeholders' support for a program, they must be able to communicate to the target population and potential stakeholders.

In addition, Health Education/Promotion Specialists must also know how to secure fiscal resources through the writing of grants as well as how to budget different resources such as money and the knowledge of health information. This is very important for health educators because money is scarce and knowing how to prioritize can lead to more effective programs.

In this area of responsibility, health educators must also be able to manage human resource aspects such as the use of effective people skills, effective leadership skills, and communication skills.

Responsibility VI: Advocacy

Health Education/Promotion Specialists take on many roles, and one of those roles is a teacher. Others will seek health advice and information from them because Health Promotion Specialists are seen as content specialists. Health Education/Promotion Specialists can be asked questions related to topics from personal health, to community-wide issues such as safety, to cancer research. Since the term "health" is so vast, it is important for the Health Education/Promotion Specialists to be aware of the available information.

While the Health Education/Promotion Specialist should be well informed, it is not essential for them to have all of the answers. When confronted with a question, it would be practically impossible to have every answer to any possible question that could be asked. However, it is more important for the Health Education/Promotion Specialist to be able to obtain the information from a credible source and relay it back to the population. There are many credible sources that can offer content that is accessible to all populations. Some sources of credible health content can be found in databases that house peer-reviewed literature, government documents, reputable organizations' websites, etc. Health Education/Promotion Specialists may even be required to develop content for specific programs and services.

Obtaining the information for the target population is important, but just as important is the Health Education/Promotion Specialists' ability to communicate the information. The dissemination of the information can range from a large target population/community to a single person. Additionally, the content can be delivered in many forms, such as face to face, through electronic portals, or even in manuscript form to reach the largest numbers in an interested population.

In many cases, the Health Education/Promotion Specialist may be working with individuals or small groups. To ensure the content has a higher likelihood of being retrieved, the Health Education/Promotion Specialist must develop a rapport with the individuals they are working with. Establishing a good relationship can help instill confidence and optimize communication. This is explained in detail in chapter 7.

Responsibility VII: Communication

In this area of responsibility, health education specialists are responsible for providing information to various groups of people from various different places and cultures. Health education specialists must stay up to date in the health field through professional development opportunities that may influence health and health education. They should be able to respond to current and future needs in health education and be able to analyze factors that influence decision-makers such as social, cultural, demographic, and political aspects.

Health educators must develop a variety of communication strategies, methods, and techniques of how to improve the health problems to distribute to the priority population. For instance, they should be able to assess the appropriateness of language in health education messages for different populations as well as be able to compare different methods of distributing educational materials. Health educators should be able to respond and communicate to the public effectively regarding health education information and be able to use culturally sensitive communication methods and techniques. Health education specialists are also responsible for promoting the health education profession individually and collectively. Specialists should also be able to advocate for individual and community health needs by initiating and supporting health legislation, rulers, policies, and procedures.

Responsibility VIII: Ethics and Professionalism

This final area of responsibility includes consistently practicing ethical principals in health educator's day to day lives. Health educators must be applying our professional code of ethics when working with any individual or community. Professional and ethical conduct should be used when planning, implementing, and evaluating health promotion programs to do this; one must use proper ethical leadership, management, and leadership. Health educators deal with sensitive topics and communities. This means that we must comply with legal standards and reporting processes. In addition to ethical guidelines, it is imperative that health educators remain professional and continue to grow in the field. For example, it is important for health educators to participate in professional associations, coalitions, and networks such as serving on committees and attending conferences.

Summary

All eight responsibilities, competencies, and sub-competencies allow health education specialists to practice their profession effectively. Health education specialists are required to have excellent skills in communication and professionalism to work with individuals and communities. As future health educators, you must be able to conduct accurate needs assessments, plan, implement, and evaluate health promotion programs. Continued study in the field of health education and health promotion is essential and necessary to stay current in our field. By becoming CHES certified or MCHES certified, you are competent in all eight areas of responsibility that are critical for effective health education to take place.

Review Questions

1. Define certification. Explain what certification is important for health educators?

2. Outline the major qualities of a certified health education specialist or health educator. What qualities do you feel like you embody?

3. Identify and discuss two ways you can stay up to date in the field of health education, health promotion, and wellness?

4. Review the eight areas of responsibility. What responsibility area do you believe you currently are the most proficient in?

Case Scenario

Sarah is a sophomore at a local university with a major in health promotion and wellness and minoring in nutrition. Sarah wants to go on to graduate school and get her MPH Master of Public Health. She is convinced she would not need to get the CHES certification because she says, "it would not do anything for her." Explain to Sarah the importance of the CHES exam. Why would it be important for Sarah to sit for the exam even though she is going on to graduate school? How could the CHES certification be beneficial for Sarah? Should Sarah sit for the exam as a Sophomore? Why or Why not?

Critical Thinking Questions

1. Knowing the characteristics of a health educator, what qualities do you think would be important for a wellness specialist? Defend why you chose these qualities.

2. After reviewing the eight areas of responsibility, was there anything missing? Are there any qualities that you believe a health educator should be responsible for or embody that are not mentioned? Why or Why not.

3. Think about the CHES exam, how could this certification benefit you in your future career path? Explain the pros and cons of the CHES exam.

Activities

1. Read the eight areas of responsibility. Create a list for each area of responsibility. Evaluate your current skills that you possess in each category. Think about the skills you wish to possess from that responsibility. Explain how you can start to work towards gaining that skillset.

2. Logon to www.NCHEC.org research the CHES exam and its requirements. Is there an exam site near where you live? Do you possess all the requirements needed to apply? How might you benefit from the CHES certification as it relates to your future?

3. Make an appointment with one of your professors that has the CHES certification. Ask them about how they studied for the exam and when they think you should take the exam. Discuss with them why they think the CHES certification is important.

Weblinks

http://www.nchec.org

National Commission for Health Education Credentialing (NCHEC)

Use this website to review the eight areas of responsibility for a health educator as well as for information regarding the CHES certification.

https://www.bls.gov/ooh/community-and-social-service/health-educators.htm

Bureau of Labor Statistics

This website provides more information about the career of health education and quick facts about health educators and community health workers.

References

American Association for Health Education (AAHE), National Commission for Health Education Credentialing (NCHEC), & Society for Public Health Education (SOPHE). (2010). Health Educator Job Analysis-2010: Executive Summary and recommendations. Retrieved June 5, 2018, from https://www.speakcdn.com/assets/2251/health_educator_job_analysis_ex_summary-final-2-19-10.pdf

Basch, C., Sliepcevich, W., Gold, R., Duncan, D., & Kolbe, L. (1985). Avoiding Type III Errors in health education program evaluations: A case study. *Health Education Quarterly, 12*(3), 315–331.

Bruening RA, Coronado F, Auld ME, Benenson G, Simone PM. (2018). Health Education Workforce: Opportunities and Challenges. *Preventing Chronic Disease (15).* doi: http://dx.doi.org/10.5888/pcd15.180045

Centers for Disease Control and Prevention. (1999). Framework for program evaluation in public health. *MMWR*; 48(No. RR-11).

Centers for Disease Control and Prevention. (2015). *Workplace health promotion: Implementation.* Retrieved from: https://www.cdc.gov/workplacehealthpromotion/model/implementation/index.html

Cleary, H. P. (1995). *The credentialing of health educators: A historical account 1970–1990.* New York: The National Commission for Health Education Credentialing, Inc.

Cottrell, R. R., Girvan, J. T. & McKenzie, J. F. (2013). *Principles & foundations of health promotion and education.* New York, NY: Benjamin Cummings.

Gilliam, A., Davis, D., Barrington, T., Lacson, R., Uhl, G., & Phoenix, U. (2002). The value of engaging stakeholders in planning and implementing evaluations. *AIDS Education and Prevention, 14*(3) [supplement], 5–17.

Green, L. W., & Lewis, F. M. (1986). *Measurement and evaluation in health education and health promotion.* Palo Alto, CA: Mayfield.

McKenzie, J. F., Neiger, B. L., & Thackeray, R. (2017) *Planning, implementing and evaluating health programs* (7th ed.). Boston: Pearson Education Inc.

McLeroy, K. R., Bibeau, D., Steckler, A., & Glanz, K. (1988). An ecological perspective on health promotion programs. *Health Education & Behavior,* 15:351–77.

National Commission for Health Education Credentialing. (2020). *Responsibilities and competencies.* Retrieved from https://www.nchec.org/responsibilities-and-competencies

National Commission for Health Education Credentialing (2018). Retrieved from https://www.nchec.org/responsibilities-and-competencies

National Task Force on the Preparation and Practice of Health Educators. (1985). *Framework for the development of competency-based curricula for entry level health educators.* New York: National Commission for Health Education Credentialing, Inc.

Salabarría-Peña, Y., Apt, B., Walsh, C. (2007). Centers for Disease Control and Prevention Developing Program Goals and Measurable Objectives from Practical Use of Program Evaluation among Sexually Transmitted Disease (STD) Programs. Retrieved May 27, 2018, from: https://www.cdc.gov/std/program/pupestd/developing%20program%20goals%20and%20objectives.pdf

Wright, J., Williams, R., & Wilkinson, J. R. (1998). Development and importance of health needs assessment. *BMJ : British Medical Journal, 316*(7140), 1310–1313.

Credits

CHAPTER 11

Various Career Venues Related to Health Promotion and Wellness

Mallory Bower

CHAPTER KEY

Authentic Learning: **using problem-solving of real-life scenarios to explore and discuss content and concepts.**

Knowledge: **the theoretical or practical understanding of a concept.**

Reflection: **contemplation or meditation.**

Practice: **applications of ideas or concepts.**

Leadership: **the act of leading a group or organization.**

Collaboration: **working with content from other organizations or peers.**

Social Justice: **fair and just relations between individuals and society.**

Chapter Objectives

- **Identify** primary career settings for health promotion and wellness (*knowledge, reflection, collaboration, and practice*).

- **Describe** the significant responsibilities of health educators within various career settings (*knowledge, reflection, collaboration, and practice*).

- **Explain** the qualifications needed for health education specialists in different careers (*knowledge, reflection, collaboration, and practice*).

- **Identify** several strategies that can be taken to help obtain a job in the field of health promotion and wellness (*knowledge, reflection, and practice*).

- **Outline** factors associated with applying to graduate schools (*knowledge, reflection, collaboration, and practice*).

- **Discuss** the need for advanced study in health promotion and wellness (*knowledge, reflection, collaboration, and practice*).

Chapter Links to the Areas of Responsibility of a Health Educator/Health Promotion Professional

- Area of Responsibility I: Assessment and Needs Capacity

- Area of Responsibility II: Planning

- Area of Responsibility V: Advocacy

- Area of Responsibility VI: Communication

- Area of Responsibility VII: Leadership Management

- Area of Responsibility VIII: Ethics and Professionalism

Introduction

There are a vast number of career opportunities related to health promotion and wellness that you can pursue. According to the Bureau of Labor Statistics (2017), job opportunities for community health workers and other health-related fields are expected to grow by 15% or more until the year 2026. The healthcare field is the largest industry in the United States today (Bureau of Labor Statistics). This chapter will provide an overview of potential career opportunities, qualifications needed for employment, and strategies for a successful job or graduate school search.

Career Opportunities and Responsibilities of Health Educators

There are several paths you can take when studying health promotion and wellness, but it is essential to understand the responsibilities of pursuing a career in this field. To help us identify specific career opportunities, we can first look at the eight major areas of responsibilities for health promotion specialists, as outlined by the NCHEC (2020):

1. Assessment of Needs Capacity

2. Planning

3. Implementation

4. Evaluation and Research

5. Advocacy

6. Communication

7. Leadership and Management

8. Ethics and Professionalism

These eight areas of responsibility for health promotion specialists can show up in many types of careers related to health promotion programming, allied health professions, and nutrition, fitness, and health administration (O*NET, 2018). For practical tips on ways to explore opportunities in the field, please refer to the *Job Search Strategies* section later in this chapter.

Careers for Health Educators and Health Promotion Specialists

A health educator and/or health promotion specialist is responsible for helping people in various populations create a lasting behavior change. Specifically, health educators/promotors perform needs analysis on specific populations, leading to the eventual planning, implementing and evaluation of these health programs. Additionally, health education/promotion specialists teach people how to manage their existing health condition with an aim and decreasing the worsening of the condition. Providing training for various health professions and advocating for improved health resources and policies to improve health also falls into the realm of a health educator. With health care moving more towards a preventative care model, there is an increased demand for health educators and/or health promotors. Instead of health care having to rely on acute-care medicine, aimed at treating a disease, instilling health educators to attempt to prevent the disease to begin with is a more viable option. For instance, creating health education programs geared at preventing obesity, instead of focusing on treating the obesity-related diseases becomes the main goal. Outlined below are only some of the different career opportunities for health educators and health promotion specialists in various venues.

School Health Education

Health educators are needed in the field of education, because they teach people about behaviors that promote wellness. In the field of education health educators are looked to for positions such as:

- **District Wellness Coordinator**: create school districts wellness policy and health initiatives, helps meet school health guidelines, evaluates overall student health.

- **Youth Program Specialist**: creates and executes health and wellness outreach plans for the youth population. Serves as an advocate for health and wellness and is responsible for youth programming related to health and wellness.

- **Head Start Health Specialist**: serves as a resource on comprehensive health services, including mental health and environmental health and safety in accordance with Head Start performance standards across the nation.

Academia and University Health Education

Health educators often find themselves teaching classes at the University level or even directing the wellness centers on college campuses. Colleges and private companies often hire health educators to develop programming aimed at decreasing the incidence of specific diseases and/or conditions. In colleges, the goal is often drug and alcohol prevention as well as mental health. Below are different jobs you may see health educators occupying within higher academia.

- **Faculty member:** Professor who is an expert in the field of health, wellness, and behavior. Teaches college students the components and skills needed to become a health educator and work in the field.

- **Health and Wellness Coordinator:** designs programs to help college students live healthier lifestyles. Provides guidance and education for improving their eight wellness dimensions.

- **Health Promotion Programmer:** creates evidence-based health promotion programs on college campuses ranging from nutrition to sexual health and much more.

- **Education Outreach Liaison:** Works collaboratively with the wellness centers on campus to provide effective outreach and education to college students that they would otherwise not receive in the classroom.

Community Health Education

Community health education focuses on promoting and protecting the health of individuals, communities and organizations.

- **Community Health Educator:** educates people about health services and develops as well as implements strategies to improve the quality of life for individuals and communities.

- **Family Services Specialist:** provides services to individuals and families such as daycare, assistance programs, food programs, affordable housing, etc.

- **Health Education Programmer:** creates programs focused on disease prevention and keeping people healthy. Develops strategies to aid in making healthy changes to one's lifestyle.

- **Community Outreach Coordinator:** oversees planning and implementation of outreach strategies for the organization or community. Cultivates relationships with the community, assesses needs, and implements the needed educational tools.

Business and Non-Profit Health Education

Many non-profit organizations will also employ health educators to create community health education programs specifically aimed at a certain population. Grant writing also plays a large role in the responsibilities of non-profit health educators.

- **Wellness Consultant:** a professional that assists individuals in achieving and maintaining optimal wellness through advisement and empowerment.

- **Health Coach:** educates and supports clients to achieve their health goals through lifestyle and behavior change.

- **Grant Writer:** responsible for preparing and creating documents to secure grant funding from the government or other foundations.

- **Cultural Competency Trainer:** a trainer that educates individuals or organizations related to value diversity, intercultural communication skills, and understanding culture.

- **Health Journalist:** a person who writes for newspapers, magazines, websites related to health and wellness information.

- **Employee Wellness Coordinator:** facilitates and directs all employees regarding health benefits and healthcare. This can include workers compensation, insurance coverages, etc.

- **Worksite Safety Coordinator:** supervises the safety of company workers. Understand legal safety requirements and sets the standards for the company. Their knowledge is used to then train employees to understand proper safety and requirements.

- **Health Marketing Coordinator:** develops an annual marketing plan, creates public awareness of events, products, and works alongside the development and communications team.

- **Clinical Research Specialist:** direct activities are related to research and development such as testing, quality control, and data collection.

Government and Health Departments

Health education specialists can work in public health departments where the focus is geared towards public health campaigns and policy change. An example would be a health education specialist working for the local county health department with an emphasis on preventing the spread of communicable diseases such as COVID-19.

- **Health Officer/Director:** communicate public health information through surveillance of health information systems. Work with policymakers and healthcare providers to help control public health problems.

- **Public Health Inspector:** a professional who inspects public establishments to ensure that they meet all state, local, and federal health laws.

- **Epidemiologist:** a public health professional who investigates patterns and causes of diseases and injury.

- **Environmental Health Educator:** works with schools, nature reserves, and nonprofits to raise awareness about environmental issues and how to live sustainably.

- **Health Information Specialist:** responsible for taking patient information and assigning codes for medical procedures.

- **Prevention Specialist:** educate at-risk youth or other populations about high risk activities such as substance abuse, violence, sexual behaviors, etc. Plans and implements programs to help individuals make better health decisions.

Skills and Qualities Employers Seek in Health Educators

Graduates of health promotion and wellness programs should have a good mix of both technical and transferable skills to achieve career success. It is crucial to take stock of your skills and qualifications at several points during your education. Starting early will help you to identify essential skills gaps so you can find opportunities that will earn you the qualifications needed to land employment after graduation. One of the primary responsibilities of a health educator is to encourage and assist individuals in adopting healthy behaviors (O*NET, 2018). Employers expect some core competencies and skill sets from their prospective employees, such as technical skills and transferable skills.

Technical Skills

Technical skills are knowledge and abilities that relate specifically to the health promotion and wellness industry. When applying for jobs, candidates will need to meet the minimum technical skills as outlined by the job description. Almost 60% of employers expect candidates to exhibit expertise and technical ability in their field, and the majority of employers cite that relevant internship experience greatly influences their hiring decisions (NACE, 2018).

Technical skills can be tied to the seven major areas of responsibilities outlined earlier in the chapter. For example, a candidate for a workplace wellness coordinator position should have completed related coursework in kinesiology, human body systems, exercise physiology and prescription, health promotion programming, essential nutrition, and perhaps even human resources. Also, competitive candidates will have practical research, work, or internship experience that is related to their academic and career goals.

Transferable Skills

In addition to academic knowledge in the area of health promotion and wellness, employers look for several other **transferable skills**. Transferable skills, sometimes referred to as "soft skills," are competencies that can be applied across careers in any industry or setting. These can be learned in the classroom, at internships and part-time jobs, or even in social settings. For example, the top three skills employers seek from college graduates across the board are teamwork, problem-solving, and communication skills (NACE, 2018). Other transferable skills include leadership, taking the initiative, analytical skills, being adaptable to change, and other qualities outlined in **Table 11.1**.

Table 11.1 ATTRIBUTES EMPLOYERS SEEK ON A CANDIDATE'S RESUME (NACE 2018)

Problem-solving Skills	Detail-oriented	Strategic Planning Skills
Ability to work in a team	Flexibility/adaptability	Creativity
Communication skills	Technical skills	Friendly/outgoing personality
Leadership	Interpersonal skills	Tactfulness
Strong work ethic	Computer skills	Entrepreneurial skills/risk-taker
Analytical/quantitative skills	Organization ability	Fluency in a foreign language
Initiative		

Copyright © 2018 by National Association of Colleges and Employers.

Job Search Strategies

Job searching can be very overwhelming and time-consuming, especially if you are taking classes and completing internships concurrently. Starting early and making a timeline (**Figure 11.1**) will undoubtedly help to keep the process manageable. Many college career services offices provide one-on-one career coaching for students (and sometimes alumni) who need help getting started and want to create a timeline that works with their career goals.

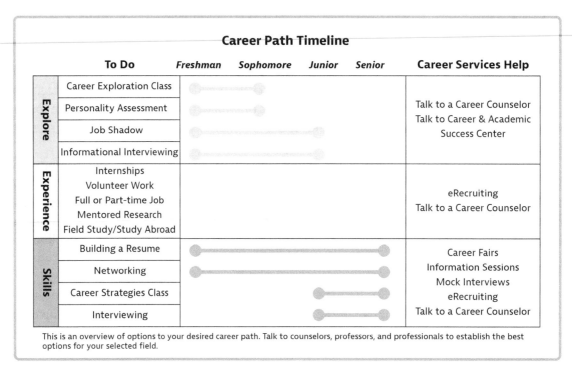

Career Path Timeline

	To Do	Freshman	Sophomore	Junior	Senior	Career Services Help
Explore	Career Exploration Class					Talk to a Career Counselor
	Personality Assessment					Talk to Career & Academic Success Center
	Job Shadow					
	Informational Interviewing					
Experience	Internships Volunteer Work Full or Part-time Job Mentored Research Field Study/Study Abroad					eRecruiting Talk to a Career Counselor
Skills	Building a Resume					Career Fairs
	Networking					Information Sessions
	Career Strategies Class					Mock Interviews eRecruiting
	Interviewing					Talk to a Career Counselor

This is an overview of options to your desired career path. Talk to counselors, professors, and professionals to establish the best options for your selected field.

Figure 11.1 *Career Exploration Timeline.*

Self-Assessment and Exploring Career Options

Knowing where to begin is half the battle. It is easy to become overwhelmed by the number of career opportunities that are available in the area of health promotion and wellness. Practical first steps are to assess your personality, interests, strengths, and values, and then to explore possible career options that align with what you found out about yourself.

Self-assessment is simply the process of knowing yourself. Take some time to reflect on your personality, your interests, your abilities, and your core values. You may want to ask yourself some questions like the ones in **Box 11.1**.

Many colleges offer multiple career inventories and assessments that will help guide you through the self-assessment process. Personality assessments like the Myers-Briggs Type Indicator can help you figure out how your personality type factors into your career choices.

Box 11.1 Self-Assessment Questions (Rutgers, 2018)

- What do I like to do in my spare time?
- In what areas have I received praise or recognition?
- Do I enjoy activities that relate to people, things, data, or ideas?
- Do I prefer to communicate in writing or verbally?
- Do I prefer a routine or a flexible schedule?
- Do I prefer to follow directions or pave my way?
- Do I enjoy analyzing complex issues, problems, or data?
- Do I enjoy creative activities and artistic endeavors?
- How important is work/life balance for me?

Other assessments such as Focus 2, StrengthsQuest, and the Strong Interest Inventory can help you begin to identify your strengths and skills. While these typically need to be interpreted by a certified career counselor, O*NET has a free assessment called the O*NET Interest Profiler that can help you 1) begin to identify your interests, values, and skills and 2) connect your results to potential career options: https://www.mynextmove.org/explore/ip.

After you have taken some time for self-assessment, it is time to explore possible career options in your field of study. A lack of exposure to specific career paths can leave you feeling overwhelmed and unsure of what options are available. The good news is that technology is making it easier for you to access this information from anywhere.

The *Occupational Outlook Handbook* is a resource that is curated and updated by the Bureau of Labor Statistics. A quick keyword search can yield various career options in addition to information about education and experience requirements, salary data, and job growth projections: https://www.bls.gov/ooh/home.htm. You can use terms from your self-assessments as keywords to search for career options.

The Explore Health Careers site will help you explore various traditional and nontraditional career paths in health and wellness. Some of the tools on this website will help you assess if a career in health is right for you, see where your skills and interests fit in the industry, and help you begin building a career that's right for you: https://explorehealthcareers.org/.

Candid Career is a clearinghouse of informational videos geared towards specific fields, including health and wellness. It gives you a snapshot of professionals' career paths and an insight into their day-to-day activities on the job: https://www.candidcareer.com/.

These are just a few of the tools available for career exploration. While assessing yourself and researching potential career options, be sure to keep track of what you find. The next steps will be to make connections with professionals and to gain experience in these areas. Taking these steps will help you confirm if some of these options will be a good fit for your personality and interests.

Making Professional Connections

Did you ever hear the phrase "It's not what you know, it's *who* you know?" Networking is one of the most effective ways to land a job. Getting to know professionals in your field of choice will help you gain insights into various paths, develop successful strategies, and confirm your interest. *How do I know where to find these people? What do I say?*

Conducting an information interview is an excellent way to meet new people and gather information about specific career fields. The purpose of this interview is to gain knowledge and insights from a person working in the field. This is quite different from a job interview because the goal is not to receive a job offer but to gather information and start building your professional network. If you have a chance to browse a few Candid Career videos, these are great examples of informational interviews with professionals from various fields.

Many campuses have formalized mentorship programs that match students with alumni in various fields. For example, the Alumni Sharing Knowledge program (A.S.K.) at the State University of New York at Oswego is designed to connect current students with alumni working in various career fields. Once matched, students can gather information about different career fields, shadow an alumnus on the job, have their resumes critiqued, practice interviewing, learn about possible internship opportunities, and make lasting connections.

LinkedIn is another excellent tool for connecting with professionals and alumni in your field. LinkedIn is the world's largest online professional network and has hundreds of millions of members worldwide (LinkedIn, 2015). After creating a professional online profile, you will have the ability to join discussion groups, browse profiles of health promotion professionals, reach out to alumni to request information interviews, and even apply for jobs and internships.

After gathering information through your career research and new professional connections, you are ready to begin preparing your professional documents and begin searching for internships and perhaps even full-time opportunities.

Preparing Job Search Materials

If you browse job descriptions in any career field, standard application requirements include a **resume**, **cover letter**, and **professional references.** It is essential to begin creating these documents early so you do not forget about any crucial credentials that could help you land a job in the future.

A **resume** is a 1–2-page document that summarizes your skills and qualifications related to health promotion and wellness. This should include relevant information about your academic degrees, professional certifications, experiences, and both transferable and technical skills. It may also include a snapshot of your work, leadership, and volunteer experience as well. Even if you do not have any professional experience or internships to add yet, start with what you *do* have and present what transferable skills you gained as a result.

Cover letters often accompany the resume as part of an application process. This is a formal, one-page letter that provides more information for the employer. It should answer a few significant questions: Why do you want this job/internship? Why do you want to work for this organization? Why should I hire you? What skills and experiences do you have that make you stand out from other candidates?

In addition to these written documents, you may need to provide contact information for **professional references**. Whether you are applying for an internship, job, or graduate school, you will need a few reliable people who can vouch for your character and professional abilities. References can make or break a job or graduate school search, so it is essential to choose carefully. Mentors, advisors, faculty, and supervisors who know you very well are usually good choices. Make sure you have a conversation with your references *before* you apply, so they are prepared to speak to your abilities positively and persuasively as it relates to the position.

Getting Experience

In a competitive job market, having a college degree is not enough to land the job. Employers are seeking graduates who have both academic knowledge and practical experience in their area of study (NACE, 2018). Out-of-classroom experiences that can help with skill-building include participating in campus organizations, shadowing or interviewing professionals in the field, completing an internship or co-op, and conducting research with a faculty member. As you learned earlier in this chapter, practical experiences greatly influence employers' hiring decisions (NACE, 2018).

Job shadowing is an on-the-job learning experience that allows you to spend time observing a professional in the field. Experiences can range from one day to a week, to semester-long terms. This differs from many other structured career development activities because you are strictly observing instead of participating directly in workplace activities. Students can complete job shadowing experiences as early as their first year in college. Examples in the health field?

Internships and **co-ops** are structured learning experiences that allow you to gain hands-on experience and to complete workplace projects related to health and wellness. The goal of an internship or co-op is to apply the theoretical knowledge gained in the classroom to a real-life workplace setting. Some academic programs even require that students complete an internship for academic credit. These types of opportunities are typically available to upper-level students, so the minimum educational requirements are met before practicing these skills in a professional setting.

Other hands-on experiences may include volunteer work, clinical observation hours, structured research, and involvement in student organizations. A good strategy is to have a diverse range of skills to help you shape your career goals and solidify your career choice. Plus, as you learned earlier in this chapter, employers are influenced positively by out-of-classroom experiences that demonstrate your technical and transferable skills in health education (NACE, 2018). Additionally, many graduate programs in the health field seek, and require, students who have contact hours with patients, such as most allied health programs. Starting this early in your educational career will not only give you insight into the career but put you ahead of others who may not be logging these experience hours.

Job Searching

By now, you have explored your strengths, narrowed down your career options, made professional relationships in your field, prepared your job search documents, and gained some experience. Before you begin applying for jobs, revisit all of this information so you can update your materials and update your network about your career plans. Most job opportunities are shared on job boards, through professional associations, and by word-of-mouth (Box 11.2).

Most applicants use online job boards to begin looking for job opportunities. The job search can be a bit of a numbers game: the more positions you apply for, the better your odds will be. This does not mean sending a generic resume to every company that pops up in your search. You will need to tailor each resume and cover letter to each specific job at each organization. When you are customizing your materials, underline or take note of the critical qualifications included in each job description. These keywords and experiences should be reflected in your documents somewhere. This is called keyword optimization. Keyword optimization is essential because many organizations use something called an Applicant Tracking System (ATS) to locate specific words in your application. Simply put, if your application does not include the required skills (keywords), you will receive an automatic rejection. Yes, customization will take quite a bit of time, but the more you spend on these details, the less time you will spend searching overall.

Successful candidates who make it through the ATS, have the required skills and experiences, and stand out from other candidates will usually receive an invitation to interview with the organization, and hopefully an offer. Job interviews allow the organization to get to know you and to see if you will be a good "fit" for their organization. Remember the personality assessments from earlier in the chapter? The interview will allow you to see if you are a good match for the company, its values, and the type of work you would be doing.

After each interview, make sure you send a nice, written thank-you note that reiterates your interest in the position and expresses your gratitude. Hand-written notes are a nice touch, but sending an email note is also appropriate as long as it is well written and sent promptly. Hopefully, soon after your follow-up, you will receive an offer for your first job!

Box 11.2 Online Job Search Engines

- Indeed.com
- Monster.com
- LinkedIn
- Zip Recruiter
- Snagajob
- NCHEC

Advanced Study and Applying to Graduate Schools

While there are several career options one can pursue with a bachelor's degree in wellness management, there are some jobs that require further study. Graduates of health promotion and wellness programs should never stop learning. The field is continually evolving, and its practitioners need to evolve along with it. This means staying up to date with laws and policies, technology, clinical techniques, content, and research practices.

Many students choose to achieve this by applying for graduate programs or to earn certifications that will open doors to additional career opportunities in medicine, counseling, administration, and advanced wellness management positions. Ideally, you should start researching programs for at least one year before graduation. This will give you time to make sure you meet the academic requirements and to gather materials required for the application. Remember: pursuing further study is a tremendous monetary and time commitment. It is essential to thoroughly research each type of program to make sure that it meets the needs of your career and financial goals.

Common Choices for Master's Degree Programs and Post-Secondary Certifications

Graduates who want to pursue careers in public health, policy, and administration may choose a Master of Public Health (**MPH**) or Master of Science in Public Health (**MSPH**). While both are focused on community health and public agencies, the MSPH curriculum tends to be more research-focused, and the MPH degree is geared more towards practitioners. While the MPH and MSPH degrees tend to be more recognized and prestigious in the field, other options include Master of Arts (**MA**), Master of Science (**MS**), Master of Business Administration (**MBA**) or Master of Education (**M.Ed.**) degree programs.

Some wellness and medical careers will require additional schooling, but not necessarily a master's or terminal degree. Careers in sports medicine, medical technology, and specific medical therapies require an associate degree or post-secondary certification.

- Anesthesiologist Assistant
- Cytotechnologist
- Certified Health Education Specialist (CHES)
- Genetic Counselor
- Histologist
- Home Health Aides
- Medical Geneticist
- Mental Health Counselor
- Medical Imaging Specialist
- Medical Research
- Medical Technologist
- Personal Trainer
- Radiation Therapist
- Respiratory Therapist
- Sports Medicine

For example, the Certified Health Education Specialist (**CHES**) exam is a practical choice for health promoters who want to demonstrate their knowledge of the seven areas of responsibility in health education. This can add a layer of credibility for entry-level graduates who are looking for jobs in various community settings.

Another example of a common certification is the National Association of Sports Medicine's (NASM) Certified Personal Training (**CPT**) credential. Students can study for and sit for their CPT exam while they are earning a bachelor's degree. This is an excellent option for students who want to gain some experience (and make some money) in the fitness industry while they are completing their degrees.

Professional Studies in Medicine and Healthcare

You may find yourself leaning toward a career in a more clinical setting. A professional career in medicine requires practitioners that are well-grounded in the liberal arts, social sciences, physical sciences, and natural sciences. Graduates from health promotion programs have a good foundation when it comes to knowledge and experience required to provide positive patient experiences. Still, more schooling is necessary for the following professions:

- Chiropractors (DC)
- Dentists (DMD) and Dental Surgeons (DDS)
- Medical Doctors and Physicians (DO, MD)
- Occupational Therapist (OPT)
- Physicians Assistants (PA)
- Physical Therapists (PT)
- Veterinary Medicine (DVM)
- Mental Health Counselor

Graduate Admissions Requirements

To gain acceptance into graduate programs, including those in medicine, you will need to meet the minimum requirements of the specific and program to which you are applying. This often includes particular courses with accompanying labs, a strong GPA, practical experience, a personal statement, and glowing letters of recommendation from supervisors and faculty.

In addition to these requirements, you will likely also need scores from required standardized tests (Box 11.3). If you remember taking the Standard Achievement Test (SAT) in high school, these are similar, but a bit more advanced and sometimes related to your field of choice. For example: if you are applying to medical school, you would need to score well on the Medical College Admission Test (MCAT). If you are applying to an MPH program, you will likely need to take the Graduate Record Exam (GRE), and for an MBA program, the Miller's Analogy Test (MAT).

Box 11.3 Graduate Entrance Exams

- Graduate Record Exam (GRE)
- Law School Admissions Test (LSAT)
- Medical College Admission Test (MCAT)
- Miller's Analogy Test (MAT)

Summary

As opportunities in health promotion and wellness continue to grow, you must know about various options and how to pursue them. Reviewing the responsibilities of health educators and taking some time for career exploration and self-assessment will help you to narrow down your choices in the field. Building relationships, networking, and gaining experience will set you on a path to becoming a life-long learner who is equipped for continued study and the rapid changes in the field.

Review Questions

1. Explain the difference between technical skills and transferable skills.

2. List three self- assessments that you could complete to help better determine your strengths and personality traits. How can these benefit you in your educational/career path?

3. List three resources that a student can use to research career paths available within the field of health and wellness.

4. Indicate what tools your school must help with searching for jobs in your field.

5. What are the common certifications that wellness professionals in the field may choose to obtain after graduation to enhance their profitability?

Case Scenario

You are working as an admission recruiter for your local college. You are asked to go into a different high school in the county to recruit prospective students to the University. You are speaking to a group of students who just came from their AP biology course. You start discussing the different majors and minors that are offered at the institution. You start talking about the Health Promotion major and the Nutrition Minor when several students begin to raise their hands. One student asks if she wanted to go into the field of medicine, what major would be better for her Biology or Health Promotion? How would you answer this question? What strengths could Health Promotion offer a student going into the medical field? The student follows up with a question regarding CHES and asks if she could sit for this certification while at your institution. How do you respond?

Critical Thinking Questions

1. Graduates of health promotion and wellness acquire many transferable skills that are essential to succeed as a wellness educator. What transferable skills do you feel are the most important to learn while in college? How might these skills help you in the field of health and wellness?

2. Take a moment to answer the self-assessment questions in **Figure 11.2**. What type of job do you feel might suit you the best? Why?

3. Networking can be the key to any future job. To start practicing networking, find a professional in a career path of your choice, and interview them to determine whether that career is for you. Ask questions such as: what made you pick your career path? What type of schooling and volunteer work did you have to complete? Etc.

Activities

1. **Make an appointment with your advisor** at your University or College to talk about your future. Ask about graduate schools and future career opportunities. Please speak with your advisor about the institutions they attended and all the degrees they earned. Ask your advisor about their thoughts on going into the workforce after graduation versus going on to complete a master's degree.

2. **Using the web link** https://www.princetonreview.com/grad-school-advice/application-timeline start mapping out your timeline for applying to graduate schools. Identify your top three institutions for graduate school. What are their requirements? When is their application deadline? Start to create your timeline and plan for applying to this school.

3. **Use the Clifton Strengths for Students website**: http://www.strengthsquest.com/. Take the self-assessment. What are your strengths? What are your weaknesses? If asked these questions in a job interview, how would you approach them? Lastly, what was your main take away from this self-assessment? What do you need to improve on, and why?

Weblinks

https://www.bls.gov/ooh/community-and-social-service/health-educators.htm#tab-2

Occupational Outlook Handbook

This site provides a background on the jobs, duties and education of health educators and community health workers.

https://www.focus2career.com/

Career Dimensions® Career & Education Planning Systems

Use this site to plan and achieve career success throughout your lifetime. The FOCUS 2 systems help connect you with colleges, career services agencies, college planners, high schools and libraries, and service organizations.

http://www.strengthsquest.com/

Clifton Strengths for Students

This site helps students learn why and how to improve academically using Gallup's online talent assessment and development solutions.

https://www.mynextmove.org/explore/ip
O*Net Interest Profile

This website helps students find out what their interests are and how they relate to the world of work. This site can also help you find out what type of career you wish to pursue.

https://explorehealthcareers.org/

Explore Health Careers: Make Your Career

Explore Health Careers is a collaboration website between today's health professionals and leading health care associations. This site uses the latest tools to guide and prepare you for a future in health care.

http://www.buzzfile.com/

The Most Advanced Company Information Database

Students can discover, research, and network with thousands of potential employers for 150+ majors.

https://www.candidcareer.com/

Candid Career

Honest career information through video. This site helps with career planning through the unique use of interviewing and narrative videos.

https://www.bls.gov/ooh/home

Occupational Outlook Handbook

This site helps guide students through a variety of jobs, different careers, and job venues. An excellent search engine tool to see what types of career paths are available.

https://www.princetonreview.com/grad-school-advice/application-timeline

Graduate School Application Timeline

If you are planning on applying to graduate school, this is the website for you! From GRE timelines and preparation guidelines, this website takes you through all the necessary steps.

https://www.nchec.org/ches

CHES Exam Eligibility

Guidelines and eligibility requirements for the Certified Health Education Specialist Exam.

https://www.nchec.org/mches

Guidelines and eligibility requirements for the Master Certified Health Education Specialist credentials.

References

Bureau of Labor Statistics. (2017). Employment Projections. Retrieved from https://www.bls.gov/emp/

Bureau of Labor Statistics. (2017). Occupational employment statistics. Retrieved from https://www.bls.gov/oes/

LinkedIn. (2015). *How LinkedIn can help you*. Retrieved from: https://www.linkedin.com/help/linkedin/answer/45/how-linkedin-can-help-you?lang=en

National Association of Colleges and Employers. (2017). *The attributes employers seek on a candidate's resume*. Retrieved from http://www.naceweb.org/talent-acquisition/candidate-selection/the-attributes-employers-seek-on-a-candidates-resume/

National Association of Colleges and Employers (NACE). (2018). *Job Outlook 2018*.

National Commission for Health Education Credentialing. (2020). *Responsibilities and competencies*. Retrieved from https://www.nchec.org/responsibilities-and-competencies

O*NET. (2018). *Online summary report for community health workers*. Retrieved from https://www.onetonline.org/link/summary/21-1094.00

Rutgers. (2018). *Guide to self-assessment*. Retrieved from https://careers.rutgers.edu/students-alumni/discover-yourself/explore-your-interests-values/guide-self-assessment

Credit

Fig. 11.1: Source: http://cougarcareerconnections.blogspot.com/2012/01/normal-0-false-false-false-en-us-x-none.html.

APPENDIX A

Code of Ethics for the Health Education Profession Preamble

The Health Education profession is dedicated to excellence in the practice of promoting individual, family, group, organizational, and community health. Guided by common goals to improve the human condition, Health Educators are responsible for upholding the integrity and ethics of the profession as they face the daily challenges of making decisions. Health Educators value diversity in society and embrace a multiplicity of approaches in their work to support the worth, dignity, potential, and uniqueness of all people.

The Code of Ethics provides a framework of shared values within the professions in which Health Education is practiced. The Code of Ethics is grounded in fundamental ethical principles including: promoting justice, doing good, and avoidance of harm. The responsibility of each health educator is to aspire to the highest possible standards of conduct and to encourage the ethical behavior of all those with whom they work.

Regardless of job title, professional affiliation, work setting, or population served, Health Educators should promote and abide by these guidelines when making professional decisions.

Article I: Responsibility to the Public

A Health Educator's responsibilities are to educate, promote, maintain, and improve the health of individuals, families, groups and communities. When a conflict of issues arises among individuals, groups, organizations, agencies, or institutions, health educators must consider all issues and give priority to those that promote the health and well-being of individuals and the public while respecting both the principles of individual autonomy, human rights and equality.

> **Section 1**: Health Educators support the right of individuals to make informed decisions regarding their health, as long as such decisions pose no risk to the health of others.

> **Section 2**: Health Educators encourage actions and social policies that promote maximizing health benefits and eliminating or minimizing preventable risks and disparities for all affected parties.

Section 3: Health Educators accurately communicate the potential benefits, risks and/or consequences associated with the services and programs that they provide.

Section 4: Health Educators accept the responsibility to act on issues that can affect the health of individuals, families, groups and communities.

Section 5: Health Educators are truthful about their qualifications and the limitations of their education, expertise and experience in providing services consistent with their respective level of professional competence.

Section 6: Health Educators are ethically bound to respect, assure, and protect the privacy, confidentiality, and dignity of individuals.

Section 7: Health Educators actively involve individuals, groups, and communities in the entire educational process in an effort to maximize the understanding and personal responsibilities of those who may be affected.

Section 8: Health Educators respect and acknowledge the rights of others to hold diverse values, attitudes, and opinions.

Article II: Responsibility to the Profession

Health Educators are responsible for their professional behavior, for the reputation of their profession, and for promoting ethical conduct among their colleagues.

Section 1: Health Educators maintain, improve, and expand their professional competence through continued study and education; membership, participation, and leadership in professional organizations; and involvement in issues related to the health of the public.

Section 2: Health Educators model and encourage nondiscriminatory standards of behavior in their interactions with others.

Section 3: Health Educators encourage and accept responsible critical discourse to protect and enhance the profession.

Section 4: Health Educators contribute to the profession by refining existing and developing new practices, and by sharing the outcomes of their work.

Section 5: Health Educators are aware of real and perceived professional conflicts of interest, and promote transparency of conflicts.

Section 6: Health Educators give appropriate recognition to others for their professional contributions and achievements

Section 7: Health educators openly communicate to colleagues, employers and professional organizations when they suspect unethical practice that violates the profession's Code of Ethics

Article III: Responsibility to Employers

Health Educators recognize the boundaries of their professional competence and are accountable for their professional activities and actions.

Section 1: Health Educators accurately represent their qualifications and the qualifications of others whom they recommend.

Section 2: Health Educators use and apply current evidence-based standards, theories, and guidelines as criteria when carrying out their professional responsibilities.

Section 3: Health Educators accurately represent potential and actual service and program outcomes to employers.

Section 4: Health Educators anticipate and disclose competing commitments, conflicts of interest, and endorsement of products.

Section 5: Health Educators acknowledge and openly communicate to employers, expectations of job-related assignments that conflict with their professional ethics.

Section 6: Health Educators maintain competence in their areas of professional practice.

Section 7: Health Educators exercise fiduciary responsibility and transparency in allocating resources associated with their work.

Article IV: Responsibility in the Delivery of Health Education

Health Educators deliver health education with integrity. They respect the rights, dignity, confidentiality, and worth of all people by adapting strategies and methods to the needs of diverse populations and communities.

Section 1: Health Educators are sensitive to social and cultural diversity and are in accord with the law, when planning and implementing programs.

Section 2: Health Educators remain informed of the latest advances in health education theory, research, and practice.

Section 3: Health educators use strategies and methods that are grounded in and contribute to the development of professional standards, theories, guidelines, data and experience.

Section 4: Health Educators are committed to rigorous evaluation of both program effectiveness and the methods used to achieve results.

Section 5: Health Educators promote the adoption of healthy lifestyles through informed choice rather than by coercion or intimidation.

Section 6: Health Educators communicate the potential outcomes of proposed services, strategies, and pending decisions to all individuals who will be affected.

Section 7: Health educators actively collaborate and communicate with professionals of various educational backgrounds and acknowledge and respect the skills and contributions of such groups.

Article V: Responsibility in Research and Evaluation

Health Educators contribute to the health of the population and to the profession through research and evaluation activities. When planning and conducting research or evaluation, health educators do so in accordance with federal and state laws and regulations, organizational and institutional policies, and professional standards.

Section 1: Health Educators adhere to principles and practices of research and evaluation that do no harm to individuals, groups, society, or the environment.

Section 2: Health Educators ensure that participation in research is voluntary and is based upon the informed consent of the participants.

Section 3: Health Educators respect and protect the privacy, rights, and dignity of research participants, and honor commitments made to those participants.

Section 4: Health Educators treat all information obtained from participants as confidential unless otherwise required by law. Participants are fully informed of the disclosure procedures.

Section 5: Health Educators take credit, including authorship, only for work they have actually performed and give appropriate credit to the contributions of others.

Section 6: Health Educators who serve as research or evaluation consultants maintain confidentiality of results unless permission is granted or in order to protect the health and safety of others.

Section 7: Health Educators report the results of their research and evaluation objectively, accurately, and in a timely fashion to effectively foster the translation of research into practice.

Section 8: Health Educators openly share conflicts of interest in the research, evaluation, and dissemination process.

Article VI: Responsibility in Professional Preparation

Those involved in the preparation and training of Health Educators have an obligation to accord learners the same respect and treatment given other groups by providing quality education that benefits the profession and the public.

Section 1: Health Educators select students for professional preparation programs based upon equal opportunity for all, and the individual's academic performance, abilities, and potential contribution to the profession and the public's health.

Section 2: Health Educators strive to make the educational environment and culture conducive to the health of all involved, and free from all forms of discrimination and harassment.

Section 3: Health Educators involved in professional preparation and development engage in careful planning; present material that is accurate, developmentally and culturally appropriate; provide reasonable and prompt feedback; state clear and reasonable expectations; and conduct fair assessments and prompt evaluations of learners.

Section 4: Health Educators provide objective, comprehensive, and accurate counseling to learners about career opportunities, development, and advancement, and assist learners in securing professional employment or further educational opportunities.

Section 5: Health Educators provide adequate supervision and meaningful opportunities for the professional development of learners.

Approved by the Coalition of National Health Education Organizations February 8, 2011

Task Force Members:

Michael Ballard

Brian Colwell

Suzanne Crouch

Stephen Gambescia

Mal Goldsmith, Chairperson

Marc Hiller

Adrian Lyde

Lori Phillips

Catherine Rasberry

Raymond Rodriquez

Terry Wessel

APPENDIX B

Areas of Responsibility, Competencies and Sub-Competencies for Health Education Specialist Practice Analysis II 2020 (HESPA II 2020)

The Eight Areas of Responsibility contain a comprehensive set of Competencies and Sub-competencies defining the role of the health education specialist. These Responsibilities were verified by the 2020 Health Education Specialist Practice Analysis II (HESPA II 2020) project and serve as the basis of the CHES® and MCHES® exam beginning 2021.

The Eight Areas of Responsibility for Health Education Specialists are:

Area I: Assessment of Needs and Capacity

Area II: Planning

Area III: Implementation

Area IV: Evaluation and Research

Area V: Advocacy

Area VI: Communication

Area VII: Leadership and Management

Area VIII: Ethics and Professionalism

Color Key:
Advanced—1
Advanced—2

The Sub-competencies shaded yellow and blue in the table below are advanced-level only and will not be included in the entry-level, CHES® examination. However, the advanced-level Sub-competencies will be included in the MCHES® examination.

HEALTH EDUCATION SPECIALIST PRACTICE ANALYSIS II 2020 (HESPA II 2020)

Competencies and Sub-Competencies

Area I: Assessment of Needs and Capacity

1.1	**Plan assessment.**
1.1.1	Define the purpose and scope of the assessment.
1.1.2	Identify priority population(s).
1.1.3	Identify existing and available resources, policies, programs, practices, and interventions.
1.1.4	Examine the factors and determinants that influence the assessment process.
1.1.5	Recruit and/or engage priority population(s), partners, and stakeholders to participate throughout all steps in the assessment, planning, implementation, and evaluation processes.

1.2	**Obtain primary data, secondary data, and other evidence-informed sources.**
1.2.1	Identify primary data, secondary data, and evidence-informed resources.
1.2.2	Establish collaborative relationships and agreements that facilitate access to data.
1.2.3	Conduct a literature review.
1.2.4	Procure secondary data.
1.2.5	Determine the validity and reliability of the secondary data.
1.2.6	Identify data gaps.
1.2.7	Determine primary data collection needs, instruments, methods, and procedures.
1.2.8	Adhere to established procedures to collect data.
1.2.9	Develop a data analysis plan.

1.3	**Analyze the data to determine the health of the priority population(s) and the factors that influence health.**
1.3.1	Determine the health status of the priority population(s).
1.3.2	Determine the knowledge, attitudes, beliefs, skills, and behaviors that impact the health and health literacy of the priority population(s).

(Continued)

HEALTH EDUCATION SPECIALIST PRACTICE ANALYSIS II 2020 (HESPA II 2020)

Competencies and Sub-Competencies (*Continued*)

Area I: Assessment of Needs and Capacity

1.3.3	Identify the social, cultural, economic, political, and environmental factors that impact the health and/or learning processes of the priority population(s).
1.3.4	Assess existing and available resources, policies, programs, practices, and interventions.
1.3.5	Determine the capacity (available resources, policies, programs, practices, and interventions) to improve and/or maintain health.
1.3.6	List the needs of the priority population(s).

1.4   Synthesize assessment findings to inform the planning process.

1.4.1	Compare findings to norms, existing data, and other information.
1.4.2	Prioritize health education and promotion needs.
1.4.3	Summarize the capacity of priority population(s) to meet the needs of the priority population(s).
1.4.4	Develop recommendations based on findings.
1.4.5	Report assessment findings.

Area II: Planning

2.1   Engage priority populations, partners, and stakeholders for participation in the planning process.

2.1.1	Convene priority populations, partners, and stakeholders.
2.1.2	Facilitate collaborative efforts among priority populations, partners, and stakeholders.
2.1.3	Establish the rationale for the intervention.

2.2   Define desired outcomes.

2.2.1	Identify desired outcomes using the needs and capacity assessment.
2.2.2	Elicit input from priority populations, partners, and stakeholders regarding desired outcomes.
2.2.3	Develop vision, mission, and goal statements for the intervention(s).
2.2.4	Develop specific, measurable, achievable, realistic, and time-bound (SMART) objectives.

2.3   Determine health education and promotion interventions.

2.3.1	Select planning model(s) for health education and promotion.
2.3.2	Create a logic model.
2.3.3	Assess the effectiveness and alignment of existing interventions to desired outcomes.
2.3.4	Adopt, adapt, and/or develop tailored intervention(s) for priority population(s) to achieve desired outcomes.
2.3.5	Plan for acquisition of required tools and resources.
2.3.6	Conduct a pilot test of intervention(s).

(Continued)

HEALTH EDUCATION SPECIALIST PRACTICE ANALYSIS II 2020 (HESPA II 2020)

Competencies and Sub-Competencies (*Continued*)

Area II: Planning

2.3.7	Revise intervention(s) based on pilot feedback.
2.4	**Develop plans and materials for implementation and evaluations.**
2.4.1	Develop an implementation plan inclusive of logic model, work plan, responsible parties, timeline, marketing, and communication.
2.4.2	Develop materials needed for implementation.
2.4.3	Address factors that influence implementation.
2.4.4	Plan for evaluation and dissemination of results.
2.4.5	Plan for sustainability.

Area III: Implementation

3.1	**Coordinate the delivery of intervention(s) consistent with the implementation plan.**
3.1.1	Secure implementation resources.
3.1.2	Arrange for implementation services.
3.1.3	Comply with contractual obligations.
3.1.4	Establish training protocol.
3.1.5	Train staff and volunteers to ensure fidelity.
3.2	**Deliver health education and promotion interventions.**
3.2.1	Create an environment conducive to learning.
3.2.2	Collect baseline data.
3.2.3	Implement a marketing plan.
3.2.4	Deliver health education and promotion as designed.
3.2.5	Employ an appropriate variety of instructional methodologies.
3.3	**Monitor implementation.**
3.3.1	Monitor progress in accordance with the timeline.
3.3.2	Assess progress in achieving objectives.
3.3.3	Modify interventions as needed to meet individual needs.
3.3.4	Ensure plan is implemented with fidelity.
3.3.5	Monitor use of resources.
3.3.6	Evaluate the sustainability of implementation.

(Continued)

HEALTH EDUCATION SPECIALIST PRACTICE ANALYSIS II 2020 (HESPA II 2020)

Competencies and Sub-Competencies (*Continued*)

Area IV: Evaluation and Research

4.1	**Design process, impact, and outcome evaluation of the intervention.**
4.1.1	Align the evaluation plan with the intervention goals and objectives.
4.1.2	Comply with institutional requirements for evaluation.
4.1.3	Use a logic model and/or theory for evaluations.
4.1.4	Assess capacity to conduct evaluation.
4.1.5	Select an evaluation design model and the types of data to be collected.
4.1.6	Develop a sampling plan and procedures for data collection, management, and security.
4.1.7	Select quantitative and qualitative tools consistent with assumptions and data requirements.
4.1.8	Adopt or modify existing instruments for collecting data.
4.1.9	Develop instruments for collecting data.
4.1.10	Implement a pilot test to refine data collection instruments and procedures.
4.2	**Design research studies.**
4.2.1	Determine purpose, hypotheses, and questions.
4.2.2	Comply with institutional and/or IRB requirements for research.
4.2.3	Use a logic model and/or theory for research.
4.2.4	Assess capacity to conduct research.
4.2.5	Select a research design model and the types of data to be collected.
4.2.6	Develop a sampling plan and procedures for data collection, management, and security.
4.2.7	Select quantitative and qualitative tools consistent with assumptions and data requirements.
4.2.8	Adopt, adapt, and/or develop instruments for collecting data.
4.2.9	Implement a pilot test to refine and validate data collection instruments and procedures.
4.3	**Manage the collection and analysis of evaluation and/or research data using appropriate technology.**
4.3.1	Train data collectors.
4.3.2	Implement data collection procedures.
4.3.3	Use appropriate modalities to collect and manage data.
4.3.4	Monitor data collection procedures.
4.3.5	Prepare data for analysis.
4.3.6	Analyze data.

(Continued)

HEALTH EDUCATION SPECIALIST PRACTICE ANALYSIS II 2020 (HESPA II 2020)

Competencies and Sub-Competencies (*Continued*)

Area IV: Evaluation and Research

4.4	Interpret data.
4.4.1	Explain how findings address the questions and/or hypotheses.
4.4.2	Compare findings to other evaluations or studies.
4.4.3	Identify limitations and delimitations of findings.
4.4.4	Draw conclusions based on findings.
4.4.5	Identify implications for practice.
4.4.6	Synthesize findings.
4.4.7	Develop recommendations based on findings.
4.4.8	Evaluate feasibility of implementing recommendations.

4.5	Use findings.
4.5.1	Communicate findings by preparing reports, and presentations, and by other means.
4.5.2	Disseminate findings.
4.5.3	Identify recommendations for quality improvement.
4.5.4	Translate findings into practice and interventions.

Area V: Advocacy

5.1	Identify a current or emerging health issue requiring policy, systems, or environmental change.
5.1.1	Examine the determinants of health and their underlying causes (e.g., poverty, trauma, and population-based discrimination) related to identified health issues.
5.1.2	Examine evidence-informed findings related to identified health issues and desired changes.
5.1.3	Identify factors that facilitate and/or hinder advocacy efforts (e.g., amount of evidence to prove the issue, potential for partnerships, political readiness, organizational experience or risk, and feasibility of success).
5.1.4	Write specific, measurable, achievable, realistic, and time-bound (SMART) advocacy objective(s).
5.1.5	Identify existing coalition(s) or stakeholders that can be engaged in advocacy efforts.

5.2	Engage coalitions and stakeholders in addressing the health issue and planning advocacy efforts.
5.2.1	Identify existing coalitions and stakeholders that favor and oppose the proposed policy, system, or environmental change and their reasons.
5.2.2	Identify factors that influence decision-makers (e.g., societal and cultural norms, financial considerations, upcoming elections, and voting record).
5.2.3	Create formal and/or informal alliances, task forces, and coalitions to address the proposed change.
5.2.4	Educate stakeholders on the health issue and the proposed policy, system, or environmental change.

(Continued)

HEALTH EDUCATION SPECIALIST PRACTICE ANALYSIS II 2020 (HESPA II 2020)

Competencies and Sub-Competencies (*Continued*)

Area V: Advocacy

5.2.5	Identify available resources and gaps (e.g., financial, personnel, information, and data).
5.2.6	Identify organizational policies and procedures and federal, state, and local laws that pertain to the advocacy efforts.
5.2.7	Develop persuasive messages and materials (e.g., briefs, resolutions, and fact sheets) to communicate the policy, system, or environmental change.
5.2.8	Specify strategies, a timeline, and roles and responsibilities to address the proposed policy, system, or environmental change (e.g., develop ongoing relationships with decision makers and stakeholders, use social media, register others to vote, and seek political appointment).

5.3	**Engage in advocacy.**
5.3.1	Use media to conduct advocacy (e.g., social media, press releases, public service announcements, and op-eds).
5.3.2	Use traditional, social, and emerging technologies and methods to mobilize support for policy, system, or environmental change.
5.3.3	Sustain coalitions and stakeholder relationships to achieve and maintain policy, system, or environmental change.

5.4	**Evaluate advocacy.**
5.4.1	Conduct process, impact, and outcome evaluation of advocacy efforts.
5.4.2	Use the results of the evaluation to inform next steps.

Area VI: Communications

6.1	**Determine factors that affect communication with the identified audience(s).**
6.1.1	Segment the audience(s) to be addressed, as needed.
6.1.2	Identify the assets, needs, and characteristics of the audience(s) that affect communication and message design (e.g., literacy levels, language, culture, and cognitive and perceptual abilities).
6.1.3	Identify communication channels (e.g., social media and mass media) available to and used by the audience(s).
6.1.4	Identify environmental and other factors that affect communication (e.g., resources and the availability of Internet access).

6.2	**Determine communication objective(s) for audience(s).**
6.2.1	Describe the intended outcome of the communication (e.g., raise awareness, advocacy, behavioral change, and risk communication).
6.2.2	Write specific, measurable, achievable, realistic, and time-bound (SMART) communication objective(s).
6.2.3	Identify factors that facilitate and/or hinder the intended outcome of the communication.

(Continued)

HEALTH EDUCATION SPECIALIST PRACTICE ANALYSIS II 2020 (HESPA II 2020)

Competencies and Sub-Competencies (*Continued*)

Area VI: Communications

6.3	**Develop message(s) using communication theories and/or models.**
6.3.1	Use communications theory to develop or select communication message(s).
6.3.2	Develop persuasive communications (e.g., storytelling and program rationale).
6.3.3	Tailor message(s) for the audience(s).
6.3.4	Employ media literacy skills (e.g., identifying credible sources and balancing multiple viewpoints).
6.4	**Select methods and technologies used to deliver message(s).**
6.4.1	Differentiate the strengths and weaknesses of various communication channels and technologies (e.g., mass media, community mobilization, counseling, peer communication, information/digital technology, and apps).
6.4.2	Select communication channels and current and emerging technologies that are most appropriate for the audience(s) and message(s).
6.4.3	Develop communication aids, materials, or tools using appropriate multimedia (e.g., infographics, presentation software, brochures, and posters).
6.4.4	Assess the suitability of new and/or existing communication aids, materials, or tools for audience(s) (e.g., the CDC Clear Communication Index and the Suitability Assessment Materials (SAM).
6.4.5	Pilot test message(s) and communication aids, materials, or tools.
6.4.6	Revise communication aids, materials, or tools based on pilot results.
6.5	**Deliver the message(s) effectively using the identified media and strategies.**
6.5.1	Deliver presentation(s) tailored to the audience(s).
6.5.2	Use public speaking skills.
6.5.3	Use facilitation skills with large and/or small groups.
6.5.4	Use current and emerging communication tools and trends (e.g., social media).
6.5.5	Deliver oral and written communication that aligns with professional standards of grammar, punctuation, and style.
6.5.6	Use digital media to engage audience(s) (e.g., social media management tools and platforms).
6.6	**Evaluate communication.**
6.6.1	Conduct process and impact evaluations of communications.
6.6.2	Conduct outcome evaluations of communications.
6.6.3	Assess reach and dose of communication using tools (e.g., data mining software, social media analytics and website analytics).

(Continued)

HEALTH EDUCATION SPECIALIST PRACTICE ANALYSIS II 2020 (HESPA II 2020)

Competencies and Sub-Competencies (*Continued*)

Area VII: Leadership and Management

7.1	**Coordinate relationships with partners and stakeholders (e.g., individuals, teams, coalitions, and committees).**
7.1.1	Identify potential partners and stakeholders.
7.1.2	Assess the capacity of potential partners and stakeholders.
7.1.3	Involve partners and stakeholders throughout the health education and promotion process in meaningful and sustainable ways.
7.1.4	Execute formal and informal agreements with partners and stakeholders.
7.1.5	Evaluate relationships with partners and stakeholders on an ongoing basis to make appropriate modifications.
7.2	**Prepare others to provide health education and promotion.**
7.2.1	Develop culturally responsive content.
7.2.2	Recruit individuals needed in implementation.
7.2.3	Assess training needs.
7.2.4	Plan training, including technical assistance and support.
7.2.5	Implement training.
7.2.6	Evaluate training as appropriate throughout the process.
7.3	**Manage human resources.**
7.3.1	Facilitate understanding and sensitivity for various cultures, values, and traditions.
7.3.2	Facilitate positive organizational culture and climate.
7.3.3	Develop job descriptions to meet staffing needs.
7.3.4	Recruit qualified staff (including paraprofessionals) and volunteers.
7.3.5	Evaluate performance of staff and volunteers formally and informally.
7.3.6	Provide professional development and training for staff and volunteers.
7.3.7	Facilitate the engagement and retention of staff and volunteers.
7.3.8	Apply team building and conflict resolution techniques as appropriate.
7.4	**Manage fiduciary and material resources.**
7.4.1	Evaluate internal and external financial needs and funding sources.
7.4.2	Develop financial budgets and plans.
7.4.3	Monitor budget performance.

(Continued)

HEALTH EDUCATION SPECIALIST PRACTICE ANALYSIS II 2020 (HESPA II 2020)

Competencies and Sub-Competencies (*Continued*)

Area VII: Leadership and Management

7.4.4	Justify value of health education and promotion using economic (e.g., cost-benefit, return-on-investment, and value-on-investment) and/or other analyses.
7.4.5	Write grants and funding proposals.
7.4.6	Conduct reviews of funding and grant proposals.
7.4.7	Monitor performance and/or compliance of funding recipients.
7.4.8	Maintain up-to-date technology infrastructure.
7.4.9	Manage current and future facilities and resources (e.g., space and equipment).

7.5 Conduct strategic planning with appropriate stakeholders.

7.5.1	Facilitate the development of strategic and/or improvement plans using systems thinking to promote the mission, vision, and goal statements for health education and promotion.
7.5.2	Gain organizational acceptance for strategic and/or improvement plans.
7.5.3	Implement the strategic plan, incorporating status updates and making refinements as appropriate.

Area VIII: Ethics and Professionalism

8.1 Practice in accordance with established ethical principles.

8.1.1	Apply professional codes of ethics and ethical principles throughout assessment, planning, implementation, evaluation and research, communication, consulting, and advocacy processes.
8.1.2	Demonstrate ethical leadership, management, and behavior.
8.1.3	Comply with legal standards and regulatory guidelines in assessment, planning, implementation, evaluation and research, advocacy, management, communication, and reporting processes.
8.1.4	Promote health equity.
8.1.5	Use evidence-informed theories, models, and strategies.
8.1.6	Apply principles of cultural humility, inclusion, and diversity in all aspects of practice (e.g., Culturally and Linguistically Appropriate Services (CLAS) standards and culturally responsive pedagogy).

8.2 Serve as an authoritative resource on health education and promotion.

8.2.1	Evaluate personal and organizational capacity to provide consultation.
8.2.2	Provide expert consultation, assistance, and guidance to individuals, groups, and organizations.
8.2.3	Conduct peer reviews (e.g., manuscripts, abstracts, proposals, and tenure folios).

8.3 Engage in professional development to maintain and/or enhance proficiency.

8.3.1	Participate in professional associations, coalitions, and networks (e.g., serving on committees, attending conferences, and providing leadership).

(*Continued*)

HEALTH EDUCATION SPECIALIST PRACTICE ANALYSIS II 2020 (HESPA II 2020)

Competencies and Sub-Competencies (*Continued*)

Area VIII: Ethics and Professionalism

8.3.2	Participate in continuing education opportunities to maintain or enhance continuing competence.
8.3.3	Develop a career advancement plan.
8.3.4	Build relationships with other professionals within and outside the profession.
8.3.5	Serve as a mentor.

8.4	**Promote the health education profession to stakeholders, the public, and others.**

8.4.1	Explain the major responsibilities, contributions, and value of the health education specialist.
8.4.2	Explain the role of professional organizations and the benefits of participating in them.
8.4.3	Advocate for professional development for health education specialists.
8.4.4	Educate others about the history of the profession, its current status, and its implications for professional practice.
8.4.5	Explain the role and benefits of credentialing (e.g., individual and program).
8.4.6	Develop presentations and publications that contribute to the profession.
8.4.7	Engage in service to advance the profession.

Updated: 10/31/19

Glossary

Action Stage when an actual behavior change is being practiced.

Adjusted Rate expressed for the entire population but can be adjusted for certain characteristics such as age (age-specific).

Advocacy public or individual support directed towards changing social, environmental, and economic conditions related to health.

Affordable Care Act (ACA) signed into law by President Barack Obama. It is healthcare that expanded coverage to 31 million uninsured Americans and focuses on both prevention and prevention services (Open Congress, 2010).

Asclepius a Thessalian chief who knew the use of drugs to heal.

Autonomy states that decision-making should focus on allowing individuals to make their own decisions based on their own lives (Coggon & Miola, 2011).

Attitude Toward the Behavior refers to one's favorable or unfavorable assessments of the behavior at hand.

Barbers surgeons or dentists who had the sharpest tools and the best chairs for surgical practices.

Behavioral Capability knowledge and skills needed to influence behavior.

Behavior Change Philosophy involves the use of behavior change contracts, goal setting, and self-monitoring to help clients or individuals foster healthy habits.

Behavior Change Theories "specify the relationships among causal processes operating both within and across levels of analysis" (McLeroy, Steckler, Goodman, & Burdine, 1992, p. 3).

Behavioral Intentions motivational factors that influence behavior.

Beneficence helps guides the decision maker to do what is "right" and what is considered "good." This principle strives to achieve "good" because we all benefit from good (Chonko, 2015).

Bloodletting the withdrawal of blood to make one healthy again and was often done by leeches or a physician.

Bubonic plague (also known as the Black Plague or Black Death) is the most severe epidemic the world has ever known, with 5,000 to 10,000 deaths in a single day (Donan, 1989, p. 94).

Certification "a process by which a professional organization grants recognition to an individual who, upon completion of a competency-based curriculum, can demonstrate a predetermined standard of performance" (Clery, 1995, p. 39).

Certified Health Education Specialist (CHES) a professionally prepared individual who possesses knowledge and skills based upon theories and research to promote behavior change within individuals and communities (Bruening et al., 2018).

Chain of Infection a model that represents the spread of communicable diseases from one host to another.

Cholera an infectious disease caused by the bacterium *vibrio cholera*. It became a major threat to the health of individuals in the 1800s.

Code of Ethics adopted by organizations to assist in understanding the difference between right and wrong within that organization.

Code of Hammurabi earliest written record of public health, contains medical laws that pertained to health practices and physicians and the first known fee schedule (Rubinson & Alles, 1984).

Cognitive-Based Philosophy focuses on content and factual information.

Committed or Commitment dedicating your time and efforts to learning about and bringing about change

Communicable Disease caused by a pathogen or disease agent and can be spread from one host to another.

Community Health "is a multi-sector and multi-disciplinary collaborative enterprise that uses public health, evidence-based strategies, and other approaches to engage and work with communities in a culturally appropriate manner to optimize the health and quality of life of all persons" (Goodman, Bunnell, & Posner, 2014).

Community Level one's living and working conditions.

Community Theory refers to behavior change approaches or participation in health behavior that can be impacted by the individual aspects of an organization, such as norms and official policies.

Community Readiness Model (CRM) is a tool used to determine what stage of readiness a group of people are in to implement a program (Edwards, Jumper-Thurman, Plested, Oetting, & Swanson, 2000).

Competencies set of characteristics and skills that enable and improve the efficiency of performance of a job.

Concepts the ideas or "building blocks" behind the theory (Rimer & Glanz, 2005).

Constructs concepts that have been developed and defined for use in theory.

Contemplation when the individual does recognize there is a problem with their current behavior and is considering making a behavior change.

Coordinated School Health Programs an organized set of policies, procedures, and activities designed to protect, promote, and improve the health and well-being of pre-K through 12 students and staff, thus improving a student's ability to learn.

Coronavirus or COVID-19 a deadly illness that includes common cold symptoms and an upper respiratory infection.

Cover Letters often accompany resumes as part of an application process.

Crude Rates are expressed for a total population.

Cues to Action the daily encounters that one may experience that could remind them that they are at risk for disease (Janz & Becker, 1984).

Culture a term that refers to the average or typical facets of a group—known as their "shared ideas, values, and perceptions. These are used to make sense of our experiences and generate behavior" (Haviland, Prins, & Walrath, 2016, p. 6).

Cultural Competence the ability to understand, communicate with, and effectively interact with people across cultures.

Decision-Making Philosophy uses cases or scenarios to help individuals analyze potential solutions and develop skills to approach health-related decisions.

Deontology states that consequences do not matter.

Diffusion of Innovation Theory a stage theory that "addresses how *new* ideas, products, and social practices, spread within an organization, community, or society" (Rimer & Glanz, 2005, p. 34).

Digital Divide is a term used to describe a barrier between current technological trends and devices based on a person's socioeconomic status and geographic location.

Disability-Adjusted Life Years (DALYs) expressed as one lost year of "healthy" life or a life living without the disability (WHO, 2019).

Early Adopters quick to adopt innovation but are not the first.

Early Majority those interested in the innovation but need additional motivation to make the change.

Eclectic Health Education/Promotion Philosophy this philosophy simply identifies that health educators are resourceful and adaptable and use many different types of philosophies when working in the field.

Educational and Ecological Assessment identifying factors and behaviors that could be influencing an individual's behaviors.

Eight Dimensions of Wellness consist of occupational, emotional, spiritual, environmental, financial, physical, social, and intellectual wellness.

Emotional Wellness is a person's ability to cope with activities of daily living (ADLs) and create satisfying relationships (SAMHSA, 2016).

Enabling Factors consist of access to healthcare facilities, services, resources, providers, and transportation.

Endemic disease present in a given geographic location.

Environmental Wellness consists of occupying pleasant and stimulating environments that support one's well-being and quality of life (SAMSHA, 2016).

Epidemic disease that rises suddenly, and the number of expected cases is more than what is considered normal for that area (CDC, 2012a).

Epidemiology branch of medicine that deals with morbidity and mortality rates and control of diseases related to health.

Epidemiological Assessment analysis of data that can identify the health needs of the priority population.

Epidemiological Data data that is collected on a national, state, and local level to assist in the prevention or control of disease outbreaks.

Ethics known as the philosophical study of "right" and "wrong" or "good" and "bad."

Evaluation measuring quality or effectiveness.

Financial Wellness overall economic state of an individual.

Focus Groups like interviews but involve five to eight people at a time.

Formative Evaluation designed during the planning process and executed during the implementation process of the program.

Freeing and Functioning Philosophy uses the same ideas from the decision-making philosophy but makes it clear that the individual is free to make their own decision then.

Generalized Model teaches the basic principles of planning and evaluation for the health professions.

Genetic Information Nondiscrimination Act (GINA) prohibits genetic discrimination in health insurance and prohibits genetic discrimination in employment.

Germ Theory states that certain diseases and illnesses are caused by certain germs or infectious agents.

Global Health is considered "collaborative transnational research and action for promoting health for all" (Beaglehole & Bonita, 2010).

Goals outcomes you intend to achieve.

Health "is a dynamic state or condition that is multidimensional (i.e., physical, emotional, social, intellectual, spiritual, and occupational), a resource for living, and results from a person's interactions with and adaptation to the environment" (Joint Committee, 2012, p. 10).

Health Belief Model explains the participation in preventive health behaviors (Hochbaum, 1958; Kegeles, Kirscht, Haefner, & Rosenstock, 1965; Rosenstock, 1966, 1974).

Health Education "any combination of learning experiences designed to help individuals and communities improve their health by increasing their knowledge or influencing their attitudes" (World Health Organization, 2017b).

Health Educator provides information on health and health related issues. They can assess health training needs and plan health education programs.

Health Equity access to the social determinants of health, specifically from wealth and power.

Health Insurance Portability and Accountability Act (HIPPA) designed to provide privacy standards to protect patients' medical records and other health information provided to health plans, doctors, hospitals, and other healthcare providers.

Health Promotion "enables people to increase control over their health. It covers a wide range of social and environmental interventions that are designed to benefit and protect individual people's health and quality of life by addressing and preventing the root causes of ill health, not just focusing on treatment and cure" (World Health Organization, 2016).

Healthy People 10-year national objectives for improving the health of all Americans.

Hippocrates the founder of the Hippocratic School of Medicine. He developed the theory of disease causation and believed that health is the result of balance, where illness is the result of an imbalance among the wellness dimensions.

Holistic Health Philosophy This philosophy achieves health and quality of life by balancing three modalities (mind, body, and spirit) for a whole being.

Hygeia daughter of Asclepius who had powers to prevent disease.

Illness-Wellness Continuum shows that an individual moving more towards the right (high-level wellness) includes awareness, education, and growth. The movement to the left (premature death) includes signs of disease and disability.

Innovators adopt innovation first.

Intellectual Wellness the knowledge and skill of an individual. When evaluating one's intellectual wellness, we must look at their creativity, problem-solving, critical thinking, and motivation to expand knowledge.

Internships structured learning experiences that allow you to gain hands-on experience and complete workplace projects related to health and wellness.

Interpersonal Levels individual's social support, social networks, social norms, and the environment.

Interpersonal Level Theories theories that assume the social environment influences individuals.

Interviews the most intimate interactions that occur between two parties during data collection.

Intrapersonal Levels look at the individual's characteristics, such as knowledge, attitudes, beliefs, skills, and motivation.

Intrapersonal Level Theories theories whose constructs are based on what the individual values.

Interventions any public health effort aimed at increasing or improving quality of life for individuals and communities.

Institutional/Organizational Level looks at the educational system, one's access to healthcare and services, and social interactions.

Job Shadowing an on-the-job learning experience that allows you to spend time observing a professional in the field.

Justice the ethical decisions that we make should be consistent and justified within the scenario (Velasquez, Andre, Shanks, & Meyer, 2020).

Laggards lack interest in innovation and are in no rush to adopt.

Late Majority consists of skeptics, those not involved in the innovation but may see practical aspects of an innovation after others.

Leprosy an infectious disease that is caused by slow-growing bacteria in the nerves, skin, eyes, and lining of the nose (nasal mucosa; CDC, 2017b).

Life Expectancy a statistical measure of the average time an organism is expected to live, based on the year of its birth, its current age, and other demographic factors, including gender.

Maintenance Stage once the behavior has been practiced for more than 6 months.

Managing Emotional Stimuli strategies or tactics to deal with emotional stimuli.

Marine Hospital Service Act established in 1798, this act "represented the first prepaid medical and hospital insurance plan in the world, under the administrative supervision of what eventually became a public health agency" (Picket & Hanlon, 1990, p. 34).

Mediating intervene or intercede between different interests in society regarding health.

Medicaid   created to assist in the payment of medical bills for the poor or those of low socioeconomic status.

Medicare   created to assist in the payment of medical bills for the elderly

Miasmas Theory   vapors or "miasmas" from rotting bodies or contagion could travel in the air great distances and be inhaled and cause disease in others (Duncan, 1988).

Mission Statement   a philosophical position that conveys an organization's values or beliefs.

Model   "models draw on several theories to help people understand a specific problem in a particular setting or context" (Rimer & Glanz, 2005).

Morality   the activity of making choices and deciding, judging, justifying, and defending those actions.

Morbidity   "having a disease or a symptom of disease, or to the amount of disease within a population" (National Cancer Institute, 2018).

Mortality Rates   "the number of deaths in a certain group of people in a certain period" (National Cancer Institute, 2018).

Multicausation Disease Model   identifies the five major risk factors for chronic disease.

Needs Assessment   a systematic process for determining and addressing needs, or "gaps," between current conditions and desired conditions, or "wants."

Noncommunicable Disease or Chronic Disease   exist in an individual for a long duration of time and progress slowly (WHO, 2013).

Objectives   are set to accomplish goals and are specific and measurable.

Observational Learning   individual's beliefs based on observing others.

Observation   noting their surroundings without really being able to gain an understanding of why and how things are happening.

Occupational Wellness   one's satisfaction with the work they do (SAMHSA, 2016).

Open-mindedness   understanding that the communities and individuals you are working with will possess perspectives that differ from your own.

Optimal Wellness   understanding and maintaining all eight dimensions of wellness.

Ottawa Charter for Health Promotion   the first International Conference on Health Promotion was held in Ottawa, Canada, in November 1986. The conference was held because of the growing public health movement taking place globally. This helped shape our understanding of health promotion and practical application strategies.

Outcome Expectations   individuals' beliefs about the results of the action.

Outcome Expectancies   the value one places on a given outcome, incentives, represents the fundamental idea that most individuals will not choose to do a task when they expect to fail.

Panacea   daughter of Asclepius who had powers to treat disease.

Pandemic "an epidemic that has spread over several countries or continents, usually affecting a large number of people" (CDC, 2012b).

Pathogen a bacterium or virus that causes disease.

Perceived Barriers the obstacles that must be overcome to make a successful behavior change (Rosenstock, 1974).

Perceived Behavioral Control one's perceptions of the ease or difficulty of performing a behavior.

Perceived benefits an individual's beliefs of whether an impact is intrinsically positive or negative (Janz & Becker, 1984).

Perceived Power factors hinder the performance of a behavior and contribute to an individual's perceived behavioral control over those factors.

Perceived Seriousness how severely one believes a disease will affect them.

Perceived Susceptibility belief of how likely it is that someone will get a disease.

Perceived Threat threat of a disease to an individual.

Philodox love of opinion.

Philosophy the study of knowledge or "thinking about thinking."

Physical Immersion refers to the health promotion specialists spending time within the physical boundaries that the target population occupies, including physical interactions with individuals of the community within these spaces.

Philosophy of Symmetry consists of four of the eight wellness dimensions: physical, emotional, spiritual, and social wellness components.

Physical Wellness consists of nutrition, physical activity, and sleep (SAMHSA, 2016).

Population Health "the health outcomes of a group of individuals, including the distribution of such outcomes within the group ... the field of population health includes health outcomes, patterns of health determinants, and policies and interventions that link these two" (Kindig & Stoddart, 2003).

Precontemplation stage in the TTM when the individual has not considered making a behavior change and will not for at least 6 months (Rimer & Glanz, 2005).

PRECEDE-PROCEED the PRECEDE-PROCEED model consists of eight phases used for creating interventions.

Predisposing Factors consist of an individual's knowledge and traits such as attitudes, beliefs, values, and perceptions.

Preparation when an individual is actively preparing to make a behavior change.

Prevention to delay or stop an unfavorable event from occurring.

Primary Data collected directly from the source.

Primary Prevention intervening before health effects occur (CDC, 2017b; Canadian Association of Physicians for the Environment, 2000).

Professional Ethics known as "actions that are right and wrong in the workplace and are of public matter."

Public Health "the science of protecting and improving the health of families and communities through the promotion of healthy lifestyles, research for disease and injury prevention and detection and control of infectious diseases" (Centers for Disease Control, 2017).

Public Policy focuses on federal, state, and local policies/laws.

Rates measures "of some event, disease, or condition, concerning a unit of population, along with a specific point in time" (National Center for Health Statistics [NCHS], 2015, p. 442).

Reinforcing Factors involve rewards and feedback after the behavior change has occurred.

Relapse stepping backward in the behavior change process.

Resume a 1–2-page document that summarizes your skills and qualifications related to health promotion and wellness.

Rights as an ethical theory, is based on the rights established by society.

Secondary Data information that already exists.

Secondary Prevention focuses on reducing the prevalence or consequences related to disease and illness.

Self-Assessment simply the process of knowing yourself.

Self-Control personal regulation of goal-directed behavior.

Self-Efficacy belief in one's ability to perform a task.

Scurvy a disease resulting from a lack of vitamin C.

Shattuck's 1850 Report of Sanitary Commission of Massachusetts a report that gave insight on how to approach and solve sanitary issues and public health in Massachusetts.

Smallpox an infectious disease that is disfiguring and often deadly.

SMART Goals goals/objectives to help individuals set small goals that are realistic and can help aid in the modification of unhealthy habits.

Smith Papyri a document that appears to be a textbook on surgery, starting with clinical cases related to head injuries (Breasted, 1922).

Social Assessment defines the quality of life within the priority population.

Social Change Philosophy looks at creating social and political change that benefits the health of an individual, group, or community.

Social Context is defined as "the sociocultural forces that shape people's day-to-day experiences and that directly and indirectly affect health and behavior" (Burke, Joseph, Pasick, & Barker, 2009, p. 56S).

Socio-Ecological Approach provides an underlying concept that behavior has multiple levels of influence. This approach "emphasizes the interaction between, and the interdependence of factors within and across all levels of a health problem" (Rimer & Glanz, 2005, p. 10).

Social Learning Theory or Social Cognitive Theory focuses on rewards, punishments, and reinforcements and how these contribute to learning.

Social Media websites or applications that enable users to create and share content or to participate in social networking.

Social Norms standard behaviors and considered normative in a group of people.

Social Wellness the intrapersonal aspects of social wellness as "developing a sense of connection, belonging, and a well-developed support system" (SAMHSA, 2016).

Spiritual wellness "expanding a sense of purpose and meaning in life" (SAMHSA, 2016).

Stakeholders individuals who have vested interests in the wellbeing of the community for various reasons.

Subjective Norms beliefs about whether others approve or disapprove of the behavior, such as peers.

Summative Evaluation "any combination of measurements and judgments that permit conclusions to be drawn about impact, outcome, or benefits of a program method" (Green & Lewis, 1986, p. 336).

Surveys fundamentally a matter of asking a sample of people from a population a set of questions and using the answers to describe that population (Fowler, 2014).

Target Population a certain group of the population that share similar characteristics and is identified as the intended audience for resources.

Technical skills are knowledge and abilities that relate specifically to the health promotion and wellness industry.

Telehealth encompasses a broad variety of technologies to assist individuals in health, health education services, and public health information.

Telemedicine delivery of health care services, where distance is a critical factor, by all health care professionals using information and communication technologies for the exchange of valid information for diagnosis, treatment and prevention of disease and injuries, research and evaluation, and for the continuing education of health care providers, all in the interests of advancing the health of individuals and their communities" (WHO, 1998).

Termination Stage there is no temptation to return to the old behavior, and the individuals have 100 percent self-efficacy in the new behavior (Prochaska & Velicer, 1997).

Tertiary prevention managing the disease, illness, or injury post-diagnosis (CDC, 2017b; Canadian Association of Physicians for the Environment, 2000).

Theory "a set of concepts, definitions, and propositions that explain or predict these events or situations by illustrating the relationships between variables" (Rimer & Glanz, 2005).

Theory of Planned Behavior (TPB) predicts and explains a wide range of health behaviors and intentions.

Transferable Skills sometimes referred to as "soft skills," are competencies that can be applied across careers in any industry or setting.

Transtheoretical Theory or Stages of Change Theory a stage theory that describes individuals' motivation and readiness to change a behavior (Rimer & Glanz, 2005).

Utilitarianism determines right from wrong by focusing on outcomes and based on the premise that ethical choices should be based on their consequences.

Virtue an ethical theory that judges individuals by their character rather than by actions that may deviate from the individual's normal behavior (Chonko, 2015).

Wellness "an approach to health that focuses on balancing the many aspects, or dimensions, of a person's life through increasing the adoption of health-enhancing behaviors rather than attempting to minimize the conditions of illness" (Joint Committee, 2012, p. 10).

Wellness Philosophy looks at balancing all eight of the wellness dimensions to form a "healthy person."

Qualitative Data data that approximates and characterizes.

Quantitative Data refers to information that has to do primarily with numbers and statistics.

Quality of Life consists of the expectations of an individual or society for a good life. These expectations are guided by the values, goals, and sociocultural context in which an individual lives.

Variables the "quantitative measurement of a construct" (Rimer & Glanz, 2005).

Years of Potential Life Lost (YPLL) measures premature mortality and is calculated by subtracting a person's age at death from the current life expectancy for that year (CDC, 1991).

Index

A

Action Stage, 72
Adjusted Rate, 44
Advocacy, 101
Affordable Care Act (ACA), 35
Asclepius, 25
Attitude Toward the Behavior, 72
Autonomy, 111

B

Barbers, 26
Behavioral Capability, 74
Behavioral Intentions, 72
Behavior Change Philosophy, 100
Behavior Change Theories, 69
Beneficence, 111
Bloodletting, 26
Bubonic plague, 26

C

Certification, 121
Certified Health Education Specialist (CHES), 121
Chain of Infection, 49
Cholera, 27
Code of Ethics, 108
Code of Hammurabi, 24
Cognitive-Based Philosophy, 100
Committed or Commitment, 88
Communicable Disease, 48
Community Health, 24
community Level, 77
Community Readiness Model (CRM), 75
Community Theory, 74
Competencies, 122
Concepts, 68
Constructs, 68
Contemplation, 71
Coordinated School Health Programs, 3
Coronavirus or COVID-19, 35
Cover Letters, 142
Crude Rates, 44
Cues to Action, 71

Cultural Competence, 85
Culture, 86

D

Decision-Making Philosophy, 100
Deontology, 111
Diffusion of Innovation Theory, 74
Digital Divide, 56
Disability-Adjusted Life Years (DALYs), 45

E

Early Adopters, 75
Early Majority, 75
Eclectic Health Education/Promotion
        Philosophy, 101
Educational and Ecological Assessment, 78
Eight Dimensions of Wellness, 14
Emotional Wellness, 14
Enabling Factors, 78
Endemic, 44
Environmental Wellness, 15
Epidemic, 44
Epidemiological Assessment, 78
Epidemiological Data, 43
Epidemiology, 43
Ethics, 107
Evaluation, 126

F

Financial Wellness, 16
Focus Groups, 124
Formative Evaluation, 126
Freeing and Functioning
        Philosophy, 100

G

Generalized Model, 77
Genetic Information Nondiscrimination
        Act (GINA), 114
Germ Theory, 28
Global Health, 3
Goals, 100

H

Health, 2
Health Belief Model, 69
Health Education, 101
Health Educator, 120
Health Equity, 110
Health Insurance Portability and Accountability
    Act (HIPPA), 114
Health Promotion, 4
Healthy People, 32
Hippocrates, 25
Holistic Health Philosophy, 99
Hygeia, 25

I

Illness-Wellness Continuum, 13
Innovators, 75
Institutional/Organizational Level, 77
Intellectual Wellness, 16
Internships, 143
Interpersonal Levels, 77
Interpersonal Level Theories, 77
Interventions, 78
Interviews, 123
Intrapersonal Levels, 77
Intrapersonal Level Theories, 77

J

Job Shadowing, 143
Justice, 111

L

Laggards, 75
Late Majority, 75
Leprosy, 26
Life Expectancy, 29

M

Maintenance Stage, 72
Managing Emotional Stimuli, 74
Marine Hospital Service Act, 30
Mediating, 7
Medicaid, 31
Medicare, 31
Miasmas Theory, 27
Mission Statement, 97

Model, 68
Morality, 107
Morbidity, 44
Mortality Rates, 44
Multicausation Disease Model, 49

N

Needs Assessment, 122
Noncommunicable Disease or Chronic Disease, 49

O

Objectives, 125
Observation, 124
Observational Learning, 74
Occupational Wellness, 18
Open-mindedness, 88
Optimal Wellness, 13
Ottawa Charter for Health Promotion, 6
Outcome Expectancies, 74
Outcome Expectations, 74

P

Panacea, 25
Pandemic, 44
Pathogen, 49
Perceived Barriers, 70
Perceived Behavioral Control, 72
Perceived benefits, 70
Perceived Power, 72
Perceived Seriousness, 71
Perceived Susceptibility, 71
Perceived Threat, 71
Philodox, 97
Philosophy, 96
Philosophy of Symmetry, 99
Physical Immersion, 88
Physical Wellness, 17
Population Health, 3
PRECEDE-PROCEED, 78
Precontemplation, 88
Predisposing Factors, 78
Preparation, 72
Prevention, 47
Primary Data, 123
Primary Prevention, 47
Professional Ethics, 108
Public Health, 24
Public Policy, 77

Q

Qualitative Data, 127
Quality of Life, 46
Quantitative Data, 127

R

Rates, 44
Reinforcing Factors, 78
Relapse, 72
Resume, 142
Rights, 112

S

Scurvy, 27
Secondary Data, 123
Secondary Prevention, 48
Self-Assessment, 140
Self-Control, 74
Self-Efficacy, 72
Shattuck's 1850 Report of Sanitary
        Commission of Massachusetts, 30
Smallpox, 26
SMART Goals, 100
Smith Papyri, 24
Social Assessment, 78
Social Change Philosophy, 101
Social Context, 76
Social Learning Theory or Social
        Cognitive Theory, 69
Social Media, 57
Social Norms, 72
Social Wellness, 18
Socio-Ecological Approach, 76

Spiritual wellness, 19
Stakeholders, 85
Subjective Norms, 72
Summative Evaluation, 127
Surveys, 124

T

Target Population, 85
Technical skills, 139
Telehealth, 62
Telemedicine, 62
Termination Stage, 72
Tertiary prevention, 48
Theory, 68
Theory of Planned Behavior (TPB), 72
Transferable Skills, 139
Transtheoretical Theory or Stages of Change Theory,
        71

U

Utilitarianism, 111

V

Variables, 68
Virtue, 112

W

Wellness, 13
Wellness Philosophy, 99

Y

Years of Potential Life Lost (YPLL), 45

CPSIA information can be obtained
at www.ICGtesting.com
Printed in the USA
LVHW062316100820
662650LV00008B/9

9 781516 524952